THE PROSTATE CANCER COMPANION: YOUR ESSENTIAL TOOLKIT FOR HEALING AND HOPE

From Diagnosis to Remission, a Step-by-Step Guide to Navigating Treatment and Embracing Life

By

Dr Gerald E. Burcham

COPYRIGHT

All rights reserved. No part of this publication may be reproduced, distributed, or transmitted in any form or by any means, including photocopying, recording, or other electronic or mechanical methods, without the prior written permission of the publisher, except in the case of brief quotations embodied in critical reviews and certain other noncommercial uses permitted by copyright law.

INTRODUCTION

In the quiet corners of life, where challenges cast long shadows, there exists the profound possibility of transformation. Meet Alex, a man standing at the crossroads of uncertainty, grappling with a formidable adversary: prostate cancer. His days were veiled in a fog of questions, fears, and the daunting task of navigating a labyrinthine healthcare landscape.

One fateful day, amidst the stacks of medical literature and conflicting advice, Alex discovered a beacon of hope – a book that would become his guiding light. As he delved into its pages, he found not just information but a companion in the journey ahead. The words leapt off the paper, demystifying the complexities of prostate cancer with clarity and compassion.

Page after page, Alex unearthed a roadmap to recovery, woven with empowering strategies, expert insights, and the latest breakthroughs in medical science. The author's words resonated with him, not merely as a guide but as a mentor, gently leading him through the maze of treatment options, addressing his concerns, and instilling a newfound sense of confidence.

In the midst of uncertainty, this book became Alex's compass, pointing him toward a future not defined by illness but by resilience and triumph. Armed with knowledge, he navigated consultations with newfound clarity, engaged with his healthcare team as an informed advocate, and, step by step, reclaimed control of his life.

This is not just a book; it is a lifeline. Join Alex on this transformative journey through the pages that changed everything. As you embark on your own Odyssey, may you find solace, empowerment, and the promise of a happy ending. Welcome to a narrative where knowledge transforms, hope prevails, and victory is not just a possibility—it's a reality waiting to unfold.

Table of Contents

Introduction

- Story of Mr Alex: In Search of Recovery.
- Discovery of a Transformative Knowledge

PART A: Understanding Prostate Cancer

CHAPTER 1: Exploration of the significance of Prostate

    1.1 Anatomy and Physiology of Prostate
    1.2 The Role of Prostate in Reproductive Health

CHAPTER 2: Risk Factors in Developing Prostate Cancer.

2.1 Aging
    2.1.1 Hormonal Changes
    2.1.2 Accumulation of Genetic Changes

2.1.3 Inflammation and Cellular Damage:

2.1.4 Cellular Senescence

2.1.5 Decreased DNA Repair Mechanisms

2.1.6 Environmental Exposures Over a Lifetime

2.1.7 Genetic Predisposition

2.2. Family History and Genetic Factors

2.2.1. Hereditary Predisposition

2.2.2 Inherited Genetic Mutations

2.2.3 Lynch Syndrome

2.2.4 Polygenic Risk Score

2.2.5 Genetic Testing and Counseling

2.3. Race and Ethnicity

2.3.1 Ethnic Disparities

2.3.2 Aggressiveness and Body Composition

2.3.3 Androgen Receptor (AR) Variants

2.3.4 Socioeconomic Factors

2.3.5 Cultural and Behavioral Factors:

2.3.6 Geographic and Environmental Influences

2.3.7 Precision Medicine Approaches

2.4. Geography and Lifestyle
2.4.1 Geographical Variation in Incidence
- Regional Disparities

2.4.2 Environmental Exposures
- Dietary Habits
- Sunlight Exposure

2.4.3. Occupational and Industrial Factors
- Occupational Hazards (exposures to carcinogens)

2.4.4. Physical Activity Levels
- Sedentary Lifestyle

2.4.5 Tobacco and Alcohol Consumption:
- Tobacco Use
- Alcohol Consumption

2.4.6. Screening Practices
- Access to Screening

2.4.7 Urbanization and Industrialization
- Environmental Pollution

2.4.8 Social and Cultural Influences:
- Cultural Practices

CHAPTER 3: Unraveling the Triggers of Prostate Cancer Onset

3.1 Genetic Mutations

3.1.1. Somatic Mutations:
- Mutation in Tumor Suppressor Genes:
- Mutation in Oncogenes:

3.1.2. Germline Mutations:
- Mutation in BRCA1 and BRCA2:
- Mutation in HOXB13 Gene

3.1.3 Mutation in DNA Repair Mechanisms:
- Mutation in Mismatch Repair Genes:

3.1.4. Androgen Receptor (AR) Mutations:
- Overexpression of Androgen Receptor:
- Point Mutations in Androgen Receptor

3.1.5 Epigenetic Alterations
- Promoter Hypermethylation

3.1.6 Chromosomal Rearrangements
- TMPRSS2-ERG Fusion:

3.2 Hormonal Influences

- Definition of Testosterone:
- Roles of Testosterone:
- Normal Androgen Function:

3.2.1 Association Between Testosterone Level and Prostate Cancer

- Low Testosterone Levels
- High Testosterone Levels
- Increased Dihydrotestosterone (DHT) Level
- Abnormal Increase In Testosterone level at Old Age

3.2.2 Imbalance in estrogen levels relative to androgens

- Estrogen Receptor Activation:

3.3 Individual Variability

3.3.1 Variability in androgen metabolism and receptor.

3.4 Chronic Inflammation Induced Prostate Cancer

3.4.1 Inflammatory Mediators and Cancer Promotion

- Release of Cytokines:
- Genomic Instability
- Immune Cell Infiltration:
- Reactive Oxygen Species (ROS):

3.4.2 Inflammatory Markers and Prostate Cancer Risk

- Elevated Biomarkers:
- Association with Aggressive Cancer

3.4.3 Immunosuppression and Cancer Escape

- Immunosuppressive Environment:

3.4.4 Tumor-Promoting Signaling

3.5 Autoimmune Inflammatory Response Trigger Prostate Cancer

3.5.1 Immunosurveillance

3.5.2. Tumor Antigens:

3.5.3 Immune Response Activation:

3.5.4 Immunosuppression and Immune Evasion

3.5.5. Chronic Inflammation:

3.5.6 Immune Checkpoints

3.5.7. Immune Escape:.

3.5.8. Local Immune Response in the Prostate:

- Immunotherapy Approaches:

3.6 Bacterial Infection triggers Prostate Cancer development

- Prostate Cancer Triggers by Microbial Infection

3.6.1 Microbial Agents and sexually transmitted Infection

3.6.2 Immune Responses to Infection

3.6.3 Dysregulation of Signaling pathways

Chapter 4: Symptoms of Prostate Cancer

4.1 urinary changes

4.1.1 Difficult and Complicated Urination

- Difficulty Initiating Urination
- Urinary Frequency and Urgency
- Weak or Intermittent Stream
- Incomplete Emptying of the Bladder
- Urinary Retention

4.1.2 Painful and bloody Urine Flow

- Pain or Discomfort During Urination
- Hematuria (Blood in Urine)

- Hematospermia (Blood in Semen)
- Pelvic Pain or Discomfort
- Symptoms of Metastasis to the Bones

4.2 Significance of Blood in Urine or Semen
- Prostate Cancer
- Urinary Tract Infections
- Prostatitis
- Benign Prostatic Hyperplasia (BPH)

4.3 Early Symptoms Interventions
4.3.1 Prompt Medical Evaluation
4.3.2 Diagnostic Considerations

4.4 Pain Management Strategies
- Pharmacological Interventions
- Interventional Procedures
- Psychosocial Support
- Palliative Care
- Emotional Considerations

4.5 Symptoms of Advanced Disease

- Pelvic Pain or Discomfort:
- Lower Back Pain:
- Ejaculatory Pain:.
- Nerve Compression and Pain:
- Neurological Symptoms:
- Bone Metastases and Pain:
- Chronic Pain Syndrome
- Jaundice
- Impact on Daily Activities
- Changes in Sexual Function
- Bone Pain and Fractures
- Weight Loss and Fatigue:
- Swelling in Legs or Pelvis

PART B: CLINICAL INVESTIGATION OF PROSTATE CANCER

Chapter 5: Diagnosing Prostate Cancer

5.1 Digital Rectal Exam(DRE)
- Purpose of DRE in Prostate Cancer Diagnosis:
  - ☐ Early Detection:

☐ Baseline Assessment

5.1.1 Procedure on how to Perform Digital Rectal Exam (DRE).
- Patient Positioning:
- Gloved and Lubricated Finger
- Prostate Palpation:.

5.1.2 Assessment of Prostate Characteristics
- Size and Consistency
- Presence of Nodules or Abnormalities.

Fig. 1: Digital Rectal Examination

Fig. 2: Digital Rectal Exam Demonstration

5.1.3 DRE in Conjunction with Other Diagnostic Measures:
- PSA Test
- Imaging Studies

5.1.4 Detection of Indicators for Further Evaluation

- Abnormal Findings

5.1.5 Patient Comfort and Communication
- Open Communication
- Explanation and Education

5.1.6 Follow-Up and Decision-Making:
- Informed Decision:
- Biopsy Consideration:
- Treatment Planning

5.1.7 Continued Advances in Diagnosis
- Technological Advancements:
- Research Contributions:

5.2 Prostate-Specific Antigen (PSA) Test

5.2.1 Purpose of the PSA Test:
- Early Detection:
- Monitoring:

5.2.2. Normal PSA Levels:

- Age-Adjusted Ranges
- Baseline PSA

5.2.3. Factors Influencing PSA Levels:
- Age
- Prostate Size
- Infection or Inflammation:
- Recent Ejaculation

5.2.4. Interpreting PSA Results:
- Normal Range:
- Elevated PSA:
- Rate of Change:
- PSA Velocity and Doubling Time:

5.2.5 PSA Density
- Adjusting for Prostate Size:

5.2.6 Advancements and Future Directions
- Novel Biomarkers
- MRI and Fusion Biopsy
- Exploring Advanced Methods

5.2.7 Procedure For Estimating Prostate-Specific Antigen (PSA)
- Consultation with Healthcare Provider
- Baseline PSA Measurement
- Follow-Up Testing
- Confirmatory Procedures
- Assessment of Risk
- Monitoring After Treatment

5.3 Prostate Biopsy Procedure
- Types of Prostate Biopsies:
  - Transrectal Ultrasound (TRUS) Biopsy:
  - Transperineal Biopsy:

5.3.1 Indications for Prostate Biopsy:
- Elevated PSA Levels
- Abnormal Digital Rectal Exam (DRE)
- Monitoring Active Surveillance:

5.3.2 Preparation for Prostate Biopsies
- Patient Education and Support

- Shared Decision-Making

5.3.3 Prostate Biopsies Execution
- Anesthesia and Antibiotic Administration
- Transrectal Ultrasound (TRUS) Guidance:
- Biopsy Needle Insertion:
- Sampling Multiple Cores:
- Specimen Collection:
- Recommendations for Further Testing:
  - Imaging Studies:
  - Repeat Biopsy

5.3.4 Post-Biopsy Considerations:
- Pathology Evaluation:
- Gleason Score:
- Discussing Results:
- Post-Biopsy Care:

5.3.5 Potential Side Effects of Prostate Biopsy Procedure
- Infection
- Bleeding

- Pain and Discomfort

5.3.6 Pathological Analysis and Follow-Up

5.3.7 Interpreting Biopsy Results

- Interpretation with Gleason Score and Grading
    - ☐ Gleason Score:
    - ☐ Gleason Grading:
- Normal/Benign Results
    - ☐ Absence of Cancer Cells
- Atypical or Suspicious Result
    - ☐ Atypical Small Acinar Proliferation (ASAP)
- High-Grade Prostatic Intraepithelial Neoplasia (PIN)

5.3.8 Cancer Detection:

- Presence of Cancer Cells:
- Cancer Location and Size:
- Staging Information:
    - ☐ Tumor Stage
    - ☐ Lymph Node Involvement:
    - ☐ Multifocality

- Multifocal Cancer

5.3.9 Advancements in Biopsy Techniques:
- Multiparametric MRI Fusion Biopsy
- Liquid Biopsy

5.3.10 Post-Treatment Monitoring:
- Treatment Decision-Making:
  - Informed Treatment Choices:
- Monitoring Recurrence
- Patient Counseling:
  - Discussing Results with Patients

Chapter 6: Importance of Early Detection in Prostate Cancer.

Screening Methods for Early Detection
- PSA Test:
- Digital Rectal Exam (DRE):
- Imaging Studies:

6.1 Increased Treatment Options

6.2 Preserving Quality of Life

6.2.1. Maintaining Normal Activities and Sexual Functions:

6.2.2. Avoiding Advanced Disease Complications:

6.2.3. Enhancing Treatment Success Rates:

6.2.4 Improving Emotional Well-Being:

6.2.5. Empowering Informed Decision-Making:

6.2.6 Supporting Long-Term Quality of Life:

6.3 Improving Prognosis

6.3.1. Increased Treatment Options: Early

6.3.2. Curative Intent:

6.3.3 Reduced Risk of Metastasis:

6.3.4 Precise Staging Information:

6.3.5 Quality of Life Considerations:

6.4 Reversing Prostate Cancer at Early Detection

6.4.1. Multidisciplinary Consultation:

6.4.2. Treatment Options:

6.4.3. Surgery and Radiation Therapy:

6.4.4. Hormone Therapy:

6.4.5 Advanced Imaging Techniques:

6.4.6 Nutritional and Lifestyle Interventions:

6.4.7. Clinical Trials and Emerging Therapies:

6.4.8. Supportive Care and Emotional Well-Being:

6.4.9. Post-Treatment Monitoring:

6.5 Other Benefits of Prostate Cancer Early detection

- Shared Decision-Making:
- Risk Stratification:
- Global Impact on Cancer Burden
- Improved Survival Rates:
- Reduced Treatment Intensity:
- Minimized Spread and Metastasis:
- Cost-Effectiveness:
- Psychological Well-being:
- Community Health Impact:.

CHAPTER 7: Further Screening and Testing for Prostate Cancer

Underlying Principle of Prostate Diagnostic Procedure

- Prostate-Specific Antigen (PSA) Test
- Digital Rectal Exam (DRE)
- Multiparametric Magnetic Resonance Imaging (mpMRI)
- Genetic Testing:
- Nomograms and Risk Calculators:

7.1 An In-Depth Exploration of Prostate Health Index (phi)

7.1.1 Prostate Health Index (phi) Procedure

- Components of Prostate Health Index:

Importance of Prostate Health Index (Phi):

- Enhanced Specificity for Prostate Cancer Detection:
- Phi Risk Stratification
- Reduction of Unnecessary Biopsies

- ☐ Clinical Validity and Guidelines:
- ☐ Combining phi with Imaging Studies Enhances Detection of Prostate Cancer
- ☐ Monitoring Prostate Cancer Patients

7.1.4 Phi Considerations and Limitations

7.1.5 Patient Education and Awareness on Phi

7.2 Multiparametric Magnetic Resonance Imaging (mpMRI) in Prostate Cancer Detection

7.2.1 Components of mpMRI
- T2-weighted Imaging:
- Diffusion-weighted Imaging (DWI):.
- Dynamic Contrast-Enhanced (DCE) Imaging:

7.2.2 Advantages of mpMRI in Prostate Cancer Detection
- ☐ Improved Localization and Visualization
- ☐ Risk Stratification
- ☐ Role in Fusion Biopsy
- ☐ Reducing Unnecessary Biopsies

- Impact on Treatment Decision-Making
- Follow-up and Monitoring
- Patient Empowerment and Informed Decision-Making

7.2.3 Considerations and Challenges

7.3 Genetic Testing for Prostate Cancer:

7.3.1. Identifying Hereditary Risk Factors: Germline and Somatic Mutations:

7.3.2 Purpose of Genetic testing in Prostate Cancer.

- Risk Stratification and Counseling:
- Familial and Inherited Patterns:
- Impact on Treatment Decision-Making:
- Early Detection and Prevention Strategies:.
- Implications for Family Members**:**

7.3.3 Challenges and Ethical Considerations

7.3.4 Future Directions in Precision Medicine

7.4 Practical Guide to Prostate Biopsy Procedures.

7.4.1. Why Biopsy is Necessary

- Confirmation of Cancer:
- Determining Grade and Stage:
- Guiding Treatment Decisions:

7.4.2. Types of Prostate Biopsy:
- Transrectal Ultrasound (TRUS) Biopsy
- Transperineal Biopsy
- MRI-Guided Biopsy

7.4.3. Preparing for a Prostate Biopsy
- Discussion with Healthcare Provider:
- Antibiotics:

   Prevention of Infection:
- Bowel Preparation:

7.4.4. During the Biopsy Procedure
- Local Anesthesia and Pain Management:
- Biopsy Needle Placement:
- Multiple Samples Collection

   Comprehensive Assessment:

7.4.5. After the Biopsy:
- Recovery Period:
- Possible Discomfort
- Pathology Analysis
- Follow-up Discussions

CHAPTER 8: Method of Classifying Prostate Cancer.

8.1. Introduction to Staging and Grading:

Staging Prostate Cancer

8.1.1 TNM Staging System:

Tumor (T):

Node (N):

Metastasis (M):

8.1.2 Grading with the Gleason Score:

Grade Group 1-5:

8.1.3 Calculating Gleason scores using Grading System

8.1.4 Impact on Treatment Decisions:

8.2 Risk Stratification of Prostate Cancer

Low, Intermediate, and High Risk Stratification:

8.2.1. Low-Risk Prostate Cancer:

a. Clinical Characteristics:

b. Prognostic Implications:

c. Treatment Considerations:

8.2.2. Intermediate-Risk Prostate Cancer:

a. **Clinical** Characteristics

b. Prognostic Implications

   c. Treatment Considerations

8.2.3. High-Risk Prostate Cancer:

   a. Clinical Characteristics:

   b. Prognostic Implications:

   c. Treatment Considerations:

8.2.4. Evolving Concepts:

a. Genomic Profiling

b. Shared Decision-Making

8.3 Clinical and Pathological Staging:

8.3.1. Clinical Staging:

a. Components of Clinical Staging

b. TNM System

c. Clinical Stage Groups

d. Limitations of Clinical Staging

8.3.2. Pathological Staging:

a. Components of Pathological Staging

b. TNM System:

c. Pathological Stage Groups:

d. Prognostic Significance:

8.3.3. Integrating Clinical and Pathological Staging

a. Multidisciplinary Assessment:

b. Post-Treatment Evaluation:

c. Advances in Imaging:

8.4. Localized and Advanced Stages of Prostate Cancer

Localized vs. Advanced Prostate Cancer:

8.4.1. Localized Prostate Cancer:

a. Criteria:

b. Diagnostic Methods:

c. Treatment Options:

Active Surveillance:

Definitive Treatments:

d. Prognosis:

8.4.2. Advanced Prostate Cancer:

a. Criteria:

b. Diagnostic Methods:

c. Treatment Options:

Systemic Therapies:

Chemotherapy:

Targeted Therapies:

d. Prognosis:

8.4.3. Transition States:

a. Biochemical Recurrence:

b. Castration-Resistant Prostate Cancer (CRPC):

8.4.4. Challenges and Advances:

a. Imaging Technologies:

b. Personalized Approaches:

PART C: Treatment for Prostate Cancer
CHAPTER 9 : Active Surveillance for Prostate Cancer
9.1 Principles of Active Surveillance

9.1.1 Rationale for Active Surveillance

Monitoring Protocols

9.2 Patient Selection Criteria

- Shared Decision-Making
- Patient Adherence and Satisfaction

9.3 Criteria for Transition to Treatment:

- Evolving Landscape
- Advancements in Monitoring Technologies:
- Integration into Multidisciplinary Care:

9.4 Psychological Aspects:

- Psychosocial Support and Education:
- Long-Term Outcomes:
- Quality of Life Considerations:

9.5 Research and Future Directions:

9.6 Facts about active surveillance

9.7 Curative Treatments for Prostate Cancer

1. Prostatectomy (Surgery):
2. Radiation Therapy:
3. Cryotherapy:
4. Hormone Therapy:
5. Focal Therapy:.

CHAPTER 10: Treatment for Prostate cancer

10.1 Prostatectomy

Introduction to Prostatectomy:

10.1.1 Types of Prostatectomy:

Radical Prostatectomy

☐ Indications for Radical Prostatectomy:

- Radical Prostatectomy Procedure:

Simple Prostatectomy:
- Indications for Simple Prostatectomy:
- Surgical Techniques:
- Simple Prostatectomy Procedure:

10.1.2 Postoperative Care:

10.1.3 Urinary Continence and Sexual

10.1.4 Follow-Up and Monitoring:

10.1.5 Advancements in Prostatectomy:

10.2 Radiation Therapy in the Treatment of Prostate Cancer:

10.2.1 Types of Radiation Therapy:
- External Beam Radiation:
- Brachytherapy:
- Proton Beam Therapy:

10.2.2. Treatment Planning and Simulation

10.2.3 Importance of Treatment Planning

10.2.4 Imaging Modalities in Treatment Planning:
- Computed Tomography (CT):.
- Magnetic Resonance Imaging (MRI):

- Positron Emission Tomography (PET):

10.2.5 . Simulation Sessions:
- **Patient Positioning**:
- **Immobilization Devices:**

10.2.6 Quality Assurance in Treatment Planning

10.2.7 Technological Advances in Treatment Planning:

Intensity-Modulated Radiation Therapy (IMRT):

Image-Guided Radiation Therapy (IGRT):

Proton Beam Therapy Planning:

10.2.8 Side Effects and Management:

10.2.9 Advances in Radiation Therapy:

10.3 HORMONE THERAPY

10.3.1 Mechanisms of Hormone Therapy:
- Androgen Deprivation:
- Prostate Cancer Cell Suppression:

Mechanisms of Hormone Therapy in the Treatment of Prostate Cancer

1. Androgen Deprivation:

a. Inhibition of Testosterone Production::

b. Blockade of Androgen Receptors:

2. Downstream Effects on Prostate Cancer Cells:

10.3.2 Indications for Hormone Therapy in the Treatment of Prostate Cancer:

10.3.3 Locally Advanced Prostate Cancer:

10.3.4. Metastatic Prostate Cancer:

a. Initial Treatment for Metastatic Disease:

b. Salvage Hormone Therapy

10.3.5. Combination Therapies:

a. Hormone Therapy with Radiation:

b. Hormone Therapy in Advanced Stages:

10.3.6 Types of Hormone Therapy in the Treatment of Prostate Cancer:

Luteinizing Hormone-Releasing Hormone (LHRH) Agonists:

LHRH Antagonists:

Anti-Androgens

10.4 IMMUNOTHERAPY

CHAPTER 11: CONCLUSION

PART A

Understanding Prostate Cancer

CHAPTER 1

Exploration of The Significance of Prostate

In the intricate tapestry of the male reproductive system, the prostate stands as a sentinel, often unnoticed until its significance becomes paramount. This chapter opens with a detailed exploration of the prostate's anatomy, function, and its pivotal role in male health. From the walnut-sized gland's location to its intricate network of ducts and muscles, we delve into the foundation of understanding this organ.

The prostate is a walnut-sized gland located just below the bladder and in front of the rectum in males. It plays a crucial role in the male reproductive system, contributing to the production of seminal fluid that nourishes and transports sperm. The gland surrounds the urethra, the tube through which urine and semen exit the body, and its position allows it to influence both urinary and reproductive functions.

1.1 ANATOMY AND PHYSIOLOGY OF PROSTATE
1.1.1 Anatomy of Prostate

- **Location:** The prostate is situated in the pelvic region, surrounding the urethra and resting against the bladder. Its location allows it to exert pressure on the urethra, affecting urine flow and contributing to various urinary functions.

- **Structure:** The prostate is divided into several zones, with the peripheral zone being the most significant concerning prostate cancer. The glandular tissue of the prostate is composed of small glands and ducts, which produce and store the prostatic fluid.

- **Blood and Nerve Supply:** The prostate receives its blood supply primarily from the inferior vesical artery. Nerves from the autonomic nervous system control the gland, influencing functions such as ejaculation.

1.1.2 Physiology of Prostate

- **Seminal Fluid Production:** The primary function of the prostate is to produce seminal fluid, a milky substance that makes up a significant portion of semen. This fluid provides nutrients, protection, and a suitable environment for sperm to survive and function optimally.

- **Muscular Contractions**: During ejaculation, smooth muscle tissue within the prostate contracts to propel the prostatic fluid into the urethra. This action, combined with contractions from other reproductive organs, facilitates the expulsion of semen from the penis.

- **Influence on Urination:** The prostate's position around the urethra means that changes in its size can affect urinary function. Conditions like benign prostatic hyperplasia (BPH) can cause the gland to enlarge, leading to symptoms such as difficulty urinating, frequent urination, and a weak urine stream.

- **Hormonal Regulation:** The prostate's growth and function are influenced by hormones, particularly testosterone and dihydrotestosterone (DHT). Imbalances in these hormones can contribute to conditions like prostate cancer.

Understanding the anatomy and physiology of the prostate is vital for comprehending its role in male reproductive and urinary health, as well as for addressing various medical conditions that may affect this important gland.

1.2 THE ROLE OF PROSTATE IN REPRODUCTIVE HEALTH.

The prostate plays a crucial role in male reproductive health by contributing to the production of seminal fluid, a key component of semen. Seminal fluid is essential for the transportation, nourishment, and protection of sperm as they journey through the male and female reproductive tracts. Here's an in-depth look at the role of the prostate in reproductive health:

1. Seminal Fluid Production: The primary function of the prostate is to produce seminal fluid, which constitutes a significant portion of semen. Seminal fluid is rich in nutrients, enzymes, and other substances that support and enhance the functionality of sperm.

2. Nutrient Supply for Sperm: Seminal fluid from the prostate provides essential nutrients for sperm, including fructose, citric acid, and various enzymes. These nutrients serve to nourish and energize sperm, enhancing their motility and overall viability.

3. Buffering and Protection: The alkaline nature of prostatic fluid helps neutralize the acidic environment of the male urethra and female reproductive tract. This alkalinity provides a more favorable environment for sperm survival and function, protecting them from the harsh acidic conditions.

4. Lubrication and Facilitation of Ejaculation:

Seminal fluid acts as a lubricant, facilitating the movement of sperm through the male reproductive system and into the female reproductive tract during ejaculation. The smooth muscle contractions of the prostate, combined with those of other reproductive organs, contribute to the expulsion of semen from the penis during ejaculation.

5. Sperm Activation: Prostatic fluid contains enzymes like prostate-specific antigen (PSA) that play a role in liquefying semen. This liquefaction is essential for the release and activation of sperm, allowing them to swim freely and effectively toward the egg for fertilization.

6. Role in Fertility: The optimal composition of seminal fluid, including the contributions from the prostate, is crucial for successful fertilization. Conditions that affect the prostate, such as infections or disorders like prostatitis, can impact the quality and functionality of seminal fluid, potentially affecting fertility.

7. Prostate's Impact on Erectile Function: While not directly related to seminal fluid production, the prostate can indirectly influence erectile function. Conditions affecting the prostate, such as benign prostatic hyperplasia (BPH), may impact sexual function and, in turn, reproductive health.

Understanding the role of the prostate in reproductive health underscores its significance in male fertility and overall reproductive function. Conditions affecting the prostate can have implications on fertility, highlighting the importance of addressing prostate health in the context of male reproductive well-being. Regular check-ups and screenings can aid in the early detection and management of conditions that may impact the prostate and, consequently, reproductive health.

CHAPTER 2

RISK FACTORS IN DEVELOPING PROSTATE CANCER.

Prostate cancer is a type of cancer that develops in the prostate, a small walnut-shaped gland in men that produces seminal fluid. It is one of the most common types of cancer among men, with varying degrees of severity and progression. Gaining a comprehensive understanding of prostate cancer involves exploring its risk factors, causes, symptoms, and the diagnostic process.

Risk Factors for Prostate Cancer: Understanding Vulnerabilities

Risk factors for prostate cancer are characteristics or exposures that have been associated with an increased likelihood of developing this specific type of cancer. These factors can vary from individual to individual, and the presence of one or more risk factors does not guarantee the development of prostate cancer. It merely indicates an elevated statistical probability. Understanding these risk factors is crucial for identifying populations at higher risk and informing screening and prevention strategies.

2.1 AGING

Prostate cancer is predominantly a disease of older men. The risk of developing prostate cancer increases significantly with age, especially after the age of 50. Age-related changes in the prostate may contribute to the development of cancer. The relationship between aging and the development of prostate cancer is complex and involves multiple factors. While aging itself is not a direct cause of prostate cancer, there are several mechanisms through which the aging process may contribute to an increased risk of developing this cancer:

2.1.1 Hormonal Changes:

As men age, there is an increase in the levels of certain hormones, such as testosterone and dihydrotestosterone (DHT). While these hormones play essential roles in normal prostate function, prolonged exposure to them may contribute to the development of prostate cancer. Testosterone is converted to DHT in the prostate, and this hormone can stimulate the growth of prostate cells, potentially leading to cancerous changes.

2.1.2 Accumulation of Genetic Changes

Over time, cells in the body accumulate genetic mutations and changes. Aging is associated with an increased likelihood of DNA damage and mutations. Some of these genetic alterations may affect the regulatory mechanisms that control cell growth and division, potentially leading to uncontrolled cell growth characteristic of cancer.

2.1.3 Inflammation and Cellular Damage:

- Chronic inflammation is common in aging tissues, and the prostate is no exception. Inflammation may result from various factors, including infections, environmental exposures, or age-related changes. Prolonged inflammation can lead to cellular damage and an environment conducive to the development of cancer.

2.1.4 Cellular Senescence:

Aging is associated with cellular senescence, a state in which cells lose their ability to divide and function properly. While senescence is a protective mechanism against the development of cancer, it can also lead to an accumulation of dysfunctional cells, contributing to age-related diseases, including cancer.

2.1.5 Decreased DNA Repair Mechanisms:

- Aging is associated with a decline in the efficiency of DNA repair mechanisms. As cells age, their ability to repair DNA damage diminishes. This can result in an increased susceptibility to mutations and the accumulation of genetic changes that may promote the development of cancer.

2.1.6 Environmental Exposures Over A Lifetime

Over a lifetime, individuals may be exposed to various environmental factors that can contribute to the development of prostate cancer. These factors may include dietary choices, exposure to carcinogens, and lifestyle habits. The cumulative effect of these exposures over time can influence cancer risk.

- **Geographical Location:** Incidence rates vary globally, with higher rates in North America and Northwestern Europe. Geographical location can contribute to differences in exposure to risk factors, including lifestyle and dietary factors.

- **Lifestyle Choices:** Diet high in saturated fats, obesity and lack of physical activity (unhealthy lifestyle choices) can contribute to an increased risk of prostate cancer.

- **Occupational Exposures:** Exposure to certain occupational hazards, like cadmium or Agent Orange may be associated with an elevated risk of prostate cancer

2.1.7 Genetic Predisposition:

While aging itself is a significant risk factor, individuals with a family history of prostate cancer may have a genetic predisposition that further increases their susceptibility. Certain genetic mutations or inherited factors can contribute to an elevated risk of developing prostate cancer.

It's important to note that aging alone does not guarantee the development of prostate cancer, and many elderly men do not develop this cancer. The interplay of genetic, hormonal, and environmental factors in the context of aging contributes to an increased risk. Regular screenings, early detection, and a comprehensive understanding of individual risk factors are essential for effective prostate cancer management in aging populations.

2.2 Family History and Genetic Factors.

Prostate cancer has a complex etiology influenced by a combination of genetic, environmental, and lifestyle factors. Understanding the role of family history and genetic factors is crucial for identifying individuals at higher risk and tailoring preventive strategies. Here's a comprehensive exploration of how family history and genetic factors contribute to the risk of prostate cancer:

2.2.1 Hereditary Predisposition

Family history plays a pivotal role in prostate cancer risk, indicating a hereditary component. Individuals with a first-degree relative (father, brother) diagnosed with prostate cancer have an elevated risk, particularly if the affected relative was diagnosed at an early age.

Risk Magnitude: The risk is proportionate to the number of affected relatives and their age at diagnosis. Multiple affected relatives or an early onset of prostate cancer in family members elevate the risk further.

2.2.2 Inherited Genetic Mutations

Inherited genetic mutations, such as mutations in BRCA1, BRCA2, or Lynch syndrome and **HOXB13** genes can increase the likelihood of developing prostate cancer **and** can be passed down through families. Carriers of HOXB13 mutation may have a higher likelihood of developing prostate cancer at a younger age.

Shared Genetic Pathways with Breast Cancer: There is an observed correlation between certain genetic factors associated with breast cancer and an increased risk of prostate cancer.

Genetic Contribution: Genes like BRCA1 and BRCA2 mutations are well-known for their link to breast and ovarian cancers, also heighten the risk of prostate cancer in men. Initial linked of BRCA1 and BRCA2 to breast cancer, have been implicated in prostate cancer development as well. Shared genetic pathways suggest overlapping susceptibility factors between these cancers.

2.2.3 Lynch Syndrome:

Lynch syndrome, a hereditary condition associated with an increased risk of various cancers, including colorectal and endometrial cancers, also elevates the risk of prostate cancer. Individuals with Lynch syndrome carry mutations in mismatch repair genes, leading to an impaired ability to correct errors in DNA replication. Prostate cancer risk is increased in male carriers of Lynch syndrome.

2.2.4 Polygenic Risk Score

Recent advancements in genetic research have led to the development of polygenic risk scores (PRS), which consider multiple genetic variants collectively to assess prostate cancer risk.

Genetic Contribution: Firstly, PRS takes into account a combination of common genetic variants associated with prostate cancer, offering a more comprehensive risk assessment. Secondly, Individuals with a high PRS may have an increased lifetime risk of developing prostate cancer.

2.2.5 Genetic Testing and Counseling:

Genetic testing can provide valuable insights into an individual's inherited risk of prostate cancer, guiding personalized screening and prevention strategies.

Genetic Counseling: Genetic counseling helps individuals understand their familial risk, interpret genetic test results, and make informed decisions about surveillance and preventive measures.

Previous Cancer History: Individuals with a history of certain cancers especially bladder cancer may have an elevated risk of developing prostate cancer

Family history and genetic factors are integral components of the prostate cancer risk landscape. Recognizing the influence of hereditary predisposition, specific gene mutations, and shared genetic pathways allows for targeted interventions, personalized screening, and proactive management strategies. Genetic counseling and testing play vital roles in empowering individuals and families with the knowledge needed to navigate their unique risk profiles and make informed decisions about prostate cancer prevention and early detection.

2.3 Race and Ethnicity

African-American men have a higher incidence of prostate cancer compared to other ethnic groups. Race and ethnicity can influence the risk, with African American men having a higher likelihood, and Asian American and Hispanic/Latino men having a lower risk compared to Caucasians. The reasons for these racial disparities are not fully understood but are likely a combination of genetic and environmental factors.

Prostate cancer exhibits striking disparities in incidence, aggressiveness, and outcomes among various racial and ethnic groups. This multifaceted phenomenon is influenced by a combination of genetic, biological, socioeconomic, and healthcare access factors. Understanding the complex relationship between race, ethnicity, and prostate cancer risk is crucial for effective prevention, early detection, and intervention. Here's an in-depth exploration:

2.3.1 Ethnic Disparities

Incidence rates of prostate cancer vary significantly among racial and ethnic groups, with African American men having the highest rates globally. Caribbean men of African descent also experience elevated incidence, while Asian and Hispanic men generally have lower rates compared to Caucasians. Certain ethnic groups exhibit higher prevalence rates of specific genetic mutations associated with an increased risk of prostate cancer. Genetic contribution show that African American men have a higher incidence of prostate cancer and are more likely to have genetic mutations associated with aggressive forms of the disease. Understanding ethnic-specific genetic factors is crucial for personalized risk assessment.

2.3.2 Aggressiveness and Body Composition

Prostate cancer in African American men tends to be more aggressive, presenting at a younger age and often with higher-grade tumors. Differences in tumor biology contribute to variations in disease outcomes.

- Genetic variations, such as specific androgen receptor variants, are more prevalent in individuals of African descent and may influence tumor aggressiveness.
- Biological distinctions associated with ethnicity disparity impact disease presentation, progression, and response to treatment.

2.3.3 Androgen Receptor (AR) Variants

Variations in the androgen receptor gene, crucial for prostate cancer development, contribute to disparities in disease characteristics.

Genetic Influence:
- Specific AR variants are more common in African American men, potentially

influencing disease susceptibility and progression.
☐ These genetic variations can affect androgen receptor signaling and contribute to the development of more advanced disease.

2.3.4 Socioeconomic Factors

Socioeconomic factors, often intertwined with race and ethnicity, play a significant role in prostate cancer risk and outcomes..

Access to Healthcare:
☐ Racial and ethnic minorities, particularly African Americans and Hispanics, may face barriers to accessing timely and high-quality healthcare services.
☐ Limited access to preventive measures and early detection efforts can contribute to later-stage diagnoses.

Healthcare Utilization:

- Differences in healthcare utilization patterns may impact prostate cancer screening participation and adherence to medical recommendations.
- Socioeconomic disparities intersect with race and ethnicity, influencing access to preventive care and early detection.

2.3.5. Cultural and Behavioral Factors

Cultural attitudes, health behaviors, and healthcare-seeking patterns vary among different racial and ethnic groups, influencing prostate cancer outcomes.

Screening Participation:

Cultural beliefs and attitudes toward healthcare can impact participation in prostate cancer screening. Culturally tailored interventions are crucial to address these differences and improve screening rates.

Treatment Decision-Making:

Cultural perspectives may influence treatment decisions and adherence to recommended therapies. Understanding these cultural nuances is essential for providing patient-centered care.

2.3.6. Geographic and Environmental Influences:

Geographic and environmental factors contribute to the complexity of prostate cancer risk among diverse populations.

Environmental Exposures:
- Varied environmental exposures, including dietary habits and lifestyle factors, contribute to diverse incidence rates.
- Geographic variations in prostate cancer risk highlight the importance of environmental influences.

2.3.7. Precision Medicine Approaches:

Advancements in precision medicine aim to address the genetic and molecular heterogeneity of prostate cancer across racial and ethnic groups.

Genomic Research:
- Ongoing research focuses on identifying genetic markers and molecular subtypes specific to different racial and ethnic backgrounds.
- Precision medicine allows for personalized treatment strategies based on the unique genomic profile of the individual.

2.3 8. Public Health Interventions:

Comprehensive public health initiatives are essential to address the racial and ethnic disparities in prostate cancer.

Education and Outreach:
- Targeted education campaigns can raise awareness about prostate cancer risk factors and the importance of early detection.

- Outreach efforts should consider cultural and linguistic diversity to effectively reach diverse communities.

Access to Healthcare: Policies and interventions that improve access to healthcare, particularly for underserved populations, are critical for reducing disparities. Ensuring equitable access to screenings and treatments is paramount.

Race and ethnicity are integral components of the complex landscape of prostate cancer risk. Recognizing the multifaceted influences of genetic, biological, socioeconomic, and cultural factors is crucial for advancing equitable and effective strategies in prevention, early detection, and treatment. Ongoing research, precision medicine approaches, and targeted public health interventions are pivotal in addressing and mitigating the disparities in prostate cancer outcomes among diverse populations.

2.4 Geography and Lifestyle:

Environmental and lifestyle factors, such as diet, may influence prostate cancer risk. Studies suggest that a diet high in saturated fats and low in fruits and vegetables may contribute to an increased risk.

Geographical Location and Lifestyle as Factors in Prostate Cancer Susceptibility

Prostate cancer susceptibility is influenced by a combination of genetic, environmental, and lifestyle factors. Geographical location and lifestyle play crucial roles in shaping an individual's risk profile for developing prostate cancer. Here's a comprehensive exploration of how these factors interplay:

2.4.1. Geographical Variation in Incidence.

Prostate cancer incidence rates vary globally and are influenced by geographical factors.
- **Regional Disparities:** Certain regions, such as North America, Northwestern Europe, and Australia, exhibit higher incidence rates

compared to Asia and Africa. Geographical clustering suggests the involvement of environmental and lifestyle elements in prostate cancer risk.

2.4.2 Environmental Exposures.

Geographical differences in environmental exposures contribute to variations in prostate cancer risk.

- **Dietary Habits:** Western countries with diets rich in red meat and high-fat content have higher prostate cancer rates while Mediterranean and Asian countries, with diets emphasizing fruits, vegetables, and fish, show lower incidence rates.

- **Sunlight Exposure:** Limited exposure to sunlight and lower vitamin D levels in regions with less sunlight may influence prostate cancer risk. Vitamin D has been implicated in prostate cancer prevention, and its synthesis is influenced by sunlight exposure.

2.4.3. Occupational and Industrial Factors:

Lifestyle factors, including occupation and industrial exposures, can impact prostate cancer risk.

- **Occupational Hazards** (exposures to carcinogens)

Certain occupational exposures to carcinogens, such as cadmium, asbestos, and pesticides, have been linked to an increased risk of prostate cancer. Geographical regions with specific industrial activities may see higher rates due to occupational exposures.

2.4.4. Physical Activity Levels:

Lifestyle choices, particularly physical activity levels, are associated with prostate cancer risk

Sedentary Lifestyle: Geographical areas with higher rates of sedentary lifestyles may see increased prostate cancer risk. Regular physical activity has been linked to a lower risk of developing prostate cancer.

2.4.5. Tobacco and Alcohol Consumption

Regional variations in tobacco and alcohol consumption contribute to lifestyle-related prostate cancer risk.

- **Tobacco Use:** Regions with higher rates of tobacco use may experience increased prostate cancer risk. Tobacco contains carcinogens that can affect prostate health.

- **Alcohol Consumption:** Excessive alcohol consumption has been associated with an elevated risk of prostate cancer. Regional differences in alcohol consumption patterns may contribute to varying prostate cancer rates.

2.4.6. Screening Practices.

Geographical variations in healthcare practices, awareness and rate of medical checkup varies in different regions. Region that practice early screenings for prostate cancer influence early detection and incidence rates.

- **Access to Screening:** Regions with better access to healthcare services and higher rates of prostate cancer screening may observe higher incidence due to early detection. Conversely, areas with limited access may experience delayed diagnoses.

2.4.7 Urbanization and Industrialization:

Urban and industrial settings may introduce additional factors impacting prostate cancer susceptibility.

- **Environmental Pollution:** Urban areas with higher levels of environmental pollution may expose individuals to carcinogens linked to prostate cancer. Industrialization may contribute to pollution and occupational exposures.

2.4.8 Social and Cultural Influences:

Cultural and social factors inherent to specific geographical regions may impact lifestyle choices and healthy behaviors.

- **Cultural Practices:** Dietary habits, cultural beliefs, and health practices vary across regions and influence lifestyle factors related to prostate cancer. Cultural considerations are crucial in developing targeted prevention and education strategies.

Geographical location and lifestyle factors intricately contribute to prostate cancer susceptibility. The interplay between environmental exposures, dietary patterns, occupational hazards, and cultural influences underscores the need for region-specific approaches to prostate cancer prevention and early detection. Comprehensive public health initiatives should consider the complex interactions of geographical and lifestyle elements to address the varying risk profiles observed globally.

CHAPTER 3

Unraveling the Triggers of Prostate Cancer Onset

The exact causes of prostate cancer remain unclear, but several factors may contribute to its development:

3.1 Genetic Mutations
Genetic Mutations and Prostate Cancer: A Comprehensive Overview

Prostate cancer is a complex disease influenced by a combination of genetic, environmental, and lifestyle factors. Genetic mutations play a pivotal role in the initiation and progression of prostate cancer. Here's a detailed exploration of how genetic mutations can contribute to the development of prostate cancer:

3.1.1. Somatic Mutations: Somatic mutations occur in non-germ cells and are not inherited but acquired during an individual's lifetime.

- **Mutation in Tumor Suppressor Genes:** Mutations in tumor suppressor genes, such as TP53 and PTEN, can disable their normal functions. Loss of function in tumor suppressors allows uncontrolled cell growth and contributes to prostate cancer development.

- **Mutation in Oncogenes**: Activation of oncogenes, like MYC, through mutations can lead to uncontrolled cell division. Increased expression of oncogenes promotes the transformation of normal prostate cells into cancerous ones.

3.1.2. Germline Mutations: Germline mutations are inherited genetic changes passed from parents to offspring. Changes in certain genes may increase the risk of prostate cancer. Inherited mutations, such as those in the BRCA1 or BRCA2 genes, are associated with a higher risk

- **Mutation in BRCA1 and BRCA2:** Mutations in BRCA1 and BRCA2, well-known for their association with breast and ovarian cancers, also increase the risk of prostate cancer in men. These genes are involved in DNA repair, and mutations compromise the cell's ability to repair DNA damage.

- **Mutation in HOXB13 Gene:** Mutations in the HOXB13 gene have been linked to hereditary prostate cancer. HOXB13 is involved in regulating cell growth, and mutations may lead to abnormal cellular proliferation.

3.1.3. Mutation in DNA Repair Mechanisms

DNA repair mechanisms are essential for maintaining genomic integrity.

- **Mutation in Mismatch Repair Genes:** Mutations in mismatch repair genes, associated with Lynch syndrome, can contribute to prostate cancer risk. Impaired mismatch repair increases the likelihood of accumulating DNA errors and mutations.

3.1.4. Androgen Receptor (AR) Mutations:

Androgen receptor mutations can alter the response to androgen hormones, influencing prostate cancer growth.

- **Overexpression of Androgen Receptor:** Amplification or overexpression of the androgen receptor is observed in some prostate cancers. This enhances the sensitivity of cancer cells to androgens, promoting tumor growth.

- **Point Mutations in Androgen Receptor:** Point mutations in the androgen receptor gene may lead to changes in receptor structure, affecting its function. Altered androgen receptor signaling contributes to the progression of prostate cancer.

3.1.5 Epigenetic Alterations:

Epigenetic changes, such as DNA methylation and histone modifications, can affect gene expression without altering the underlying DNA sequence.

- **Promoter Hypermethylation:** Hypermethylation of tumor suppressor gene promoters can lead to their silencing.

- Inactivation of tumor suppressors through epigenetic changes promotes prostate cancer development.

3.1.6 Chromosomal Rearrangements

Structural changes in chromosomes, such as translocations and inversions, can result in gene fusions and alterations.

- **TMPRSS2-ERG Fusion:**
  The TMPRSS2-ERG gene fusion is a common chromosomal rearrangement in prostate cancer. This fusion can lead to overexpression of the ERG oncogene, promoting prostate cancer growth.

Genetic mutations are integral drivers of prostate cancer, influencing critical pathways involved in cell growth, DNA repair, and hormone signaling. Understanding the diverse genetic alterations associated with prostate cancer is crucial for developing targeted therapies, precision medicine approaches, and personalized treatment strategies. Research efforts continue to uncover the intricate genetic landscape of prostate cancer, paving the way for advancements in diagnosis, prognosis, and therapeutic interventions.

3.2 Hormonal Influences

Imbalances in androgen levels or abnormal androgen receptor activity can lead to uncontrolled proliferation of prostate cells.

Definition of Testosterone:

- Testosterone is a primary male sex hormone and a potent androgen. It belongs to the class of androgens and is responsible for the development of male reproductive tissues and secondary sexual characteristics.

- Androgens are a group of hormones that stimulate the development of male characteristics, such as facial hair, deep voice, and muscle growth. They are produced in both males and females.

Roles of Testosterone:

- Testosterone is primarily produced in the testes in males.
- Androgens, including testosterone, are pivotal in the development of male reproductive organs, such as the testes and prostate.
- Testosterone has a significant impact on sexual desire, erectile function, and overall sexual health in men.
- Androgens, including testosterone, contribute to the development and maintenance of muscle and bone mass.
- Testosterone, is crucial for promoting muscle growth and maintaining bone density.
- Testosterone plays a role in reducing body fat and promoting a more muscular physique in men.
- Testosterone is essential for the development of sperm and the maintenance of male fertility.

- Androgens interact with other hormones in the endocrine system to maintain hormonal balance. Likewise, testosterone interacts with estrogen, another key sex hormone, in a delicate hormonal balance in both males and females.
- Imbalances in testosterone levels can contribute to conditions such as hypogonadism, affecting reproductive and sexual health.
- Hormones, particularly testosterone, play a role in prostate cancer. Hormonal imbalances or higher levels of testosterone influence the risk of prostate cancer or changes in how the prostate responds to hormones may contribute to cancer development.

Normal Androgen Function:
1. Androgens bind to and activate the androgen receptor (AR) in prostate cells, regulating

gene expression and maintaining normal prostate function.
2. Androgens support the normal growth and proliferation of prostate cells.
3. Androgens play a physiological role in promoting the growth and development of the prostate during puberty and maintaining its function throughout adulthood.

Androgen Receptor Signaling on: Androgen receptor signaling is crucial for the growth, differentiation, and maintenance of the prostate epithelium

3.2.1 Association Between Testosterone Level and Prostate Cancer

Prostate cancer is highly influenced by hormones, particularly androgens, which include testosterone and dihydrotestosterone (DHT). The intricate relationship between hormones and prostate cancer involves multiple processes, and disruptions in this delicate balance can contribute to the development and progression of prostate cancer. Here's a comprehensive exploration of how hormones can play a role in causing prostate cancer

The relationship between testosterone levels and prostate cancer is complex and not fully understood. Historically, there has been a concern that higher levels of testosterone might contribute to an increased risk of prostate cancer due to the hormone's role in the development and maintenance of the prostate gland. However, recent research has led to a more nuanced understanding, and the relationship is not as straightforward as previously thought.

Low Testosterone Levels:
I. Some studies have suggested that lower levels of testosterone might be associated with a decreased risk of developing prostate cancer.
II. However, the evidence is not conclusive, and more research is needed to establish a

clear link between low testosterone levels and reduced prostate cancer risk.

High Testosterone Levels:
Contrary to earlier beliefs, current research does not consistently support a direct association between high testosterone levels and an increased risk of prostate cancer. It's essential to note that prostate cancer is a multifactorial disease, and hormonal influences are just one aspect of its development.

Increased Dihydrotestosterone (DHT) Level
DHT, a more potent form of testosterone, plays a significant role in prostate cancer. The conversion of testosterone to DHT is facilitated by the enzyme 5-alpha reductase. Elevated DHT levels can result in increased androgen receptor activation, contributing to prostate cancer development.

Abnormal Increase In Testosterone Level At Old Age

Age-related changes, including alterations in hormone levels, contribute to prostate cancer risk. As men age, there is a decline in testosterone levels, and the prostate may become more sensitive to lower androgen concentrations. Age-related hormonal changes can influence the development of prostate cancer. Therefore, at old age abnormal increase in testosterone may result in proliferation of the prostate cells.

Prostate cancer that depends on androgens for growth is termed hormone-sensitive or hormone-responsive. Hormone-sensitive prostate cancer cells rely on androgens for their growth and survival. Androgen deprivation therapy (ADT) is a common treatment approach to reduce androgen levels and slow cancer growth.

Therefore, Anti-androgen therapies are designed to block androgen receptor activity. Prostate cancer often initially responds well to anti-androgen therapies, leading to tumor regression. However, resistance can develop, and cancer cells may find alternative ways to activate androgen receptor signaling.

3.2.2. Imbalance in Estrogen Level Relative to Androgens

Hormonal balance, including the interplay between testosterone and other hormones like estrogen, might be more crucial than absolute testosterone levels alone. Estrogens, typically considered female hormones, also play a role in prostate cancer.

- **Estrogen Receptor Activation:** Prostate tissue contains estrogen receptors, and estrogen signaling can affect prostate cell growth. Imbalances in estrogen levels relative to androgens may contribute to prostate cancer development.

3.3 Individual Variability:

The response to testosterone can vary among individuals, and genetic factors may play a role in how the body processes and responds to hormones.

3.3.1 Variability in androgen metabolism and receptor.

Genetic factors and mutations can contribute to an imbalance in hormonal regulation. Some individuals may inherit genetic mutations that affect androgen metabolism or receptor function, increasing their susceptibility to prostate cancer. Mutations in the androgen receptor gene can alter receptor structure and function, leading to aberrant signaling and promoting cancerous growth.

Androgens, primarily testosterone and its metabolite DHT, stimulate the growth and function of the prostate gland. Abnormal androgen receptor activity can lead to uncontrolled proliferation of prostate cells.

The relationship between hormones and prostate cancer is intricate and multifaceted. While androgens are essential for normal prostate function, imbalances, genetic mutations, and age-related changes can lead to the initiation and progression of prostate cancer. Understanding these dynamics is crucial for developing targeted therapeutic approaches, including hormonal therapies, to manage and treat prostate cancer effectively. Ongoing research continues to deepen our understanding of the interplay between hormones and prostate cancer, providing insights into novel treatment strategies and personalized interventions.

3.4 Chronic Inflammation Induced Prostate Cancer

Chronic inflammation of the prostate, often a result of infections or other conditions, may be linked to an increased risk of cancer.

Chronic Inflammation of the Prostate and Its Link to Increased Cancer Risk:

Chronic inflammation of the prostate, a condition often associated with infections or other underlying conditions, has been implicated in the increased risk of developing prostate cancer. This intricate relationship involves a complex interplay of immune responses, inflammatory pathways, and potential genomic alterations. Here's an in-depth exploration of the connection between chronic prostate inflammation and heightened cancer risk:

The prostate, like any other tissue, can experience acute inflammation as a part of the body's natural immune response to infections or injuries. Persistent or chronic inflammation occurs when the immune response is prolonged, leading to sustained release of inflammatory mediators.

3.4.1 Inflammatory Mediators and Cancer Promotion:

Release of Cytokines: During chronic inflammation, cells release pro-inflammatory cytokines, such as interleukin-6 (IL-6) and tumor necrosis factor-alpha (TNF-α).

Prolonged exposure to these cytokines may create a microenvironment conducive to cancer development.

Genomic Instability: Chronic inflammation can induce genomic instability, potentially leading to DNA damage and mutations. Altered genetic material may contribute to the initiation and progression of prostate cancer.

Immune Cell Infiltration:
Immune Cells in the Prostate: In response to chronic inflammation, immune cells infiltrate the prostate tissue. Macrophages, lymphocytes, and other immune cells contribute to the inflammatory milieu.

Reactive Oxygen Species (ROS): Immune cells may produce reactive oxygen species (ROS) as part of the inflammatory response. ROS can cause oxidative stress and damage DNA, potentially promoting carcinogenesis.

3.4.2 Inflammatory Markers and Prostate Cancer Risk:

Elevated Biomarkers: Elevated levels of inflammatory markers, such as C-reactive protein (CRP), in the blood have been associated with an increased risk of prostate cancer.

Association with Aggressive Cancer: Chronic inflammation is particularly linked to the development of more aggressive forms of prostate cancer. Aggressive tumors may exhibit higher levels of inflammation-related markers.

3.4.3 Immunosuppression and Cancer Escape:

Immunosuppressive Environment: Chronic inflammation may create an immunosuppressive environment that allows cancer cells to evade the immune system's surveillance.

3.4.4 Tumor-Promoting Signaling:

Inflammatory signaling pathways can interact with tumor cells, promoting their survival, proliferation, and invasion.

Chronic inflammation of the prostate, whether triggered by infections or other conditions, emerges as a potential contributor to an increased risk of prostate cancer. The complex interplay between inflammatory responses, genomic alterations, and the tumor microenvironment underscores the need for further research to unravel the precise mechanisms linking chronic inflammation to prostate cancer. Targeting inflammation-related pathways may offer avenues for both prevention and therapeutic interventions in the context of prostate cancer.

3.5 Autoimmune Inflammatory Response Triggers Prostate Cancer

Non-infectious factors like autoimmune reactions or irritants can also contribute to chronic inflammation in the prostate

The relationship between the immune response and prostate cancer is complex and involves intricate interactions within the body. The immune system's primary function is to recognize and eliminate abnormal or potentially harmful cells, including those that could develop into cancer. However, cancer cells can sometimes evade the immune system's surveillance or create an immunosuppressive environment that allows them to proliferate. Here's a breakdown of how the immune response in the prostate may be involved in the development of cancer:

3.5.1. Immunosurveillance: The immune system constantly monitors the body for abnormal cells, including those with potential cancerous changes. Immune cells, such as T cells and natural killer (NK) cells, play a crucial role in recognizing and eliminating these abnormal cells. Macrophages, dendritic cells, and other immune cells in the prostate contribute to immune surveillance and response. The balance between pro-inflammatory and anti-inflammatory signals can influence the effectiveness of immune responses in the prostate

3.5.2. Tumor Antigens: Cancer cells often produce unique proteins or antigens that can be recognized by the immune system. Immune cells can identify these tumor antigens as foreign or abnormal and mount an immune response against them.

3.5.3. Immune Response Activation: When the immune system detects abnormal cells, it activates an immune response to destroy or control them. T cells, in particular, can recognize and target cells displaying tumor antigens.

3.5.4. Immunosuppression and Immune Evasion: Cancer cells can develop mechanisms to evade immune detection or create an immunosuppressive microenvironment. Tumor cells may produce factors that inhibit the activity of immune cells or create a protective shield against immune attack.

3.5.5. Chronic Inflammation: Chronic inflammation in the prostate may contribute to the development of cancer. Inflammatory processes can attract immune cells to the site, but persistent inflammation can create an environment conducive to cancer initiation and progression.

3.5.6. Immune Checkpoints: Some cancers, including prostate cancer, can exploit immune checkpoints to evade immune attack. Immune checkpoint proteins, such as PD-1 and PD-L1, regulate the immune response. Cancer cells may overexpress these proteins to dampen the immune response.

3.5.7. Immune Escape: Cancer cells can undergo changes that allow them to escape immune detection. This may involve mutations that alter the expression of antigens or proteins involved in immune recognition.

3.5.8. Local Immune Response in the Prostate: The prostate has its own local immune environment, and disruptions in immune surveillance mechanisms can impact cancer development. Immune cells in the prostate may be influenced by hormonal changes, genetic factors, or inflammatory signals.

Immunotherapy aims to leverage the immune system to target and destroy cancer cells. Approaches like immune checkpoint inhibitors are being explored in prostate cancer treatment to enhance the immune response against tumors.

The interplay between the immune response and prostate cancer is a dynamic and evolving field of research. Understanding the factors that influence immune surveillance, immune evasion, and the local immune environment in the prostate is crucial for developing targeted therapies and immunotherapeutic approaches. Ongoing research aims to uncover the complexities of this relationship and identify strategies to harness the immune system in the fight against prostate cancer.

3.6 Bacterial Infection triggers Prostate Cancer development:

Chronic inflammation of the prostate, often due to prostatitis may contribute to an increased risk of developing prostate cancer. Bacterial infections, such as chronic prostatitis, can trigger persistent inflammation in the prostate. Inflammatory responses to infectious agents may continue even after the infection is seemingly resolved.

Prostate Cancer Triggers by Microbial Infection

The relationship between microbial infections and the development of prostate cancer is an area of ongoing research, and the mechanisms involved are not yet fully understood. While chronic inflammation, often triggered by infections, has been linked to an increased risk of various cancers, including prostate cancer, the direct causative relationship is complex. Here's an overview of the potential connections:

3.6.1 Microbial Agents (sexually transmitted infections): Specific microbial agents, such as certain bacteria or viruses, have been studied in relation to prostate cancer. Some studies have suggested associations between certain infections (e.g., sexually transmitted infections) and an increased risk of prostate cancer.

Some studies have explored the potential role of specific infectious agents, such as the bacteria associated with prostatitis, in prostate cancer development. The evidence linking specific microbes to prostate cancer remains an area of active investigation.

Genetic factors may influence how the prostate responds to infections and inflammation. Environmental factors, including lifestyle and exposures, may also play a role in the interplay between infections and prostate cancer risk.

3.6.2 Immune Responses to Infection:

Microbial infections in the prostate can lead to chronic inflammation, which is a known risk factor for cancer development. Persistent inflammation creates an environment that may promote genetic mutations, tissue damage, and abnormal cell growth.

When the body detects an infection, the immune system responds with an inflammatory reaction to eliminate the pathogen. Chronic infections may result in sustained inflammation, increasing the release of pro-inflammatory molecules.

Inflammatory processes generate reactive oxygen species (ROS), which can cause DNA damage.

DNA damage can lead to genetic mutations that may contribute to the initiation and progression of cancer.

In response to infection and inflammation, immune cells are recruited to the site of infection in the prostate. Immune cells can release inflammatory mediators that, when chronically elevated, may contribute to tissue damage.

3.6.3 Dysregulation of signaling pathways: Chronic inflammation can lead to altered cellular signaling pathways in the prostate cells. Dysregulation of signaling pathways may promote uncontrolled cell growth and survival.

Elevated levels of inflammatory biomarkers, such as cytokines and chemokines, have been detected in the prostates of individuals with prostate cancer. These biomarkers may reflect ongoing inflammation and immune responses.

Strategies to prevent or manage chronic infections, particularly those causing prostatitis, may be considered as potential preventive measures. Proactive management of infections and inflammation could have implications for reducing prostate cancer risk.

While the association between microbial infections and prostate cancer is complex, chronic inflammation triggered by infections is a recognized factor that may contribute to the development of prostate cancer. Ongoing research aims to elucidate the specific mechanisms, identify potential infectious agents, and explore preventive and therapeutic strategies to mitigate the impact of infections on prostate health.

CHAPTER 4

Symptoms of Prostate Cancer

Symptoms of Prostate Cancer: An In-Depth Exploration

Prostate cancer, especially in its early stages, may not exhibit noticeable symptoms. As the cancer progresses, individuals may experience: urinary changes, Blood in Urine or Semen, Discomfort or pain at pelvic region during ejaculation, although these can also be indicative of non-cancerous conditions. It's crucial for individuals to be vigilant about any changes in their health and promptly seek medical evaluation if they experience the following symptoms:

It's important to note that these symptoms are not exclusive to prostate cancer and can be caused by various other conditions. Moreover, early-stage prostate cancer may be asymptomatic. Regular health check-ups, especially for individuals at higher risk, and prompt medical evaluation if symptoms arise, play a crucial role in the early detection and effective management of prostate cancer. If individuals experience persistent or concerning symptoms, consulting with a healthcare professional for appropriate evaluation and diagnostic testing is strongly recommended.

4.1. Urinary Changes as a Symptom of Prostate Cancer

- Frequent urination, especially at night

☐ Difficulty starting or stopping urination
☐ Weak or interrupted urine flow

Prostate cancer can manifest with various symptoms, and changes in urinary patterns are often among the early signs. Understanding these urinary changes is crucial for early detection and timely intervention. Here's a comprehensive exploration of the urinary symptoms associated with prostate cancer:

4.1.1 Difficult and Complicated Urination:

- **Difficulty Initiating Urination**
  Difficulty starting the urinary stream or a weak urine flow can be a symptom.
  Prostate cancer can cause obstruction of the urethra, making it difficult to start urination. Tumor growth within the prostate may

narrow the urethral passage, creating resistance against the flow of urine.

- **Urinary Frequency and Urgency.**

  Urinary Incontinence: Difficulty controlling urine flow, leading to leakage or incontinence, may occur. Individuals notice an increase in the frequency of urination, particularly during the night (nocturia), and a sense of urgency to urinate are common urinary changes. Prostate cancer, as it progresses, may obstruct the urethra, leading to irritative symptoms. The heightened urgency results from the increased pressure on the bladder.

- **Weak or Intermittent Stream**

  A weakened or intermittent urinary stream is a common symptom associated with prostate cancer. Obstruction caused by the tumor can impede the smooth flow of urine from the bladder through the urethra.

- **Incomplete Emptying of the Bladder:** Individuals with prostate cancer may experience a feeling of not completely emptying their bladder after urination. The obstructive nature of prostate cancer can hinder the efficient emptying of the bladder, leading to residual urine.

- **Urinary Retention:** In severe cases, prostate cancer can lead to urinary retention, where the individual is unable to pass urine. Complete obstruction of the urethra may prevent any urine flow, necessitating prompt medical attention.

4.1.2 Painful and bloody Urine Flow

- **Pain or Discomfort During Urination:** Pain or discomfort during urination may occur in individuals with advanced prostate cancer. Tumor growth and infiltration into adjacent structures can cause irritation and pain during the passage of urine

- **Hematuria (Blood in Urine):** In some cases, prostate cancer may lead to the presence of blood in the urine, a condition known as hematuria. And it may present as discoloration ranging from pink to dark red. Tumor invasion or irritation of the surrounding tissues can cause bleeding, resulting in the discoloration of urine my
- **Hematospermia**, hematospermia refers to the presence of blood in semen, leading to a reddish or brownish appearance. Prostate cancer can contribute to hematospermia, especially if the tumor affects the prostate's surrounding structures or seminal vesicles. Other benign conditions, such as infections, inflammation, or trauma, may also cause hematospermia.

- **Pelvic Pain or Discomfort:** Prostate cancer can be associated with pelvic pain or discomfort, often extending to the lower back. Advanced stages of prostate cancer may involve the invasion of nearby tissues, triggering pain in the pelvic and lumbar regions.
- **Symptoms of Metastasis to the Bones:** Advanced prostate cancer, when it metastasizes to the bones, can cause additional urinary symptoms. Bone metastases may lead to increased bone pain, affecting the pelvic area and potentially impacting urinary function.

4.2 Significance of Blood in Urine or Semen
- **Prostate Cancer:** Presence of blood in urine or semen can be a symptom, although it may not always indicate cancer. The presence of blood in urine or semen can be alarming and may indicate various underlying conditions, including prostate cancer. A prevalent cancer among men, prostate cancer can

develop when cells in the prostate undergo abnormal growth. Early detection through screening is crucial for effective treatment.

- **Urinary Tract Infections:** While these symptoms are not exclusive to prostate cancer, they serve as crucial signals that warrant medical attention. Significance of blood in urine also includes other non-cancerous conditions, such as urinary tract infections or kidney stones. Recurrent urinary tract infections may be a sign of an obstructed or enlarged prostate.

- **Prostatitis**: Inflammation of the prostate, often caused by infection, can result in pain and discomfort

- **Benign Prostatic Hyperplasia (BPH):** It's important to note that blood in urine or semen does not definitively indicate prostate cancer. Non-cancerous conditions, such as infections, inflammation, or benign prostatic hyperplasia (BPH), can also lead to these symptoms. Benign Prostatic Hyperplasia (BPH) is a non-cancerous enlargement of the prostate, common in aging males and can lead to urinary symptoms due to its impact on the urethra.

4.3 Early Symptoms Interventions

4.3.1 Prompt Medical Evaluation:

Timely Intervention: Individuals experiencing blood in urine or semen should seek prompt medical attention. Blood in urine or semen can serve as an early warning sign of prostate cancer, prompting further investigation by healthcare professionals.

Comprehensive evaluation, including imaging studies, blood tests, and potentially a prostate biopsy, is essential for accurate diagnosis and appropriate management. Medical evaluation, including imaging studies and cystoscopy, is crucial to identify the underlying cause of hematuria. Prostate cancer may be considered among potential causes, particularly if other symptoms or risk factors are present.

Blood in urine or semen should be regarded as a significant symptom that necessitates medical evaluation. While prostate cancer is one potential cause, a thorough diagnostic process is crucial to identify the underlying condition accurately. Early detection and timely intervention not only aid in addressing potential cancer concerns but also contribute to overall urological health and well-being. Individuals experiencing these symptoms should engage with healthcare professionals for a comprehensive assessment and personalized care.

Urinary changes serve as significant indicators of prostate cancer, reflecting the impact of tumor growth on the urinary system. Monitoring and recognizing these symptoms, especially in the context of age and risk factors, enable individuals to seek timely medical attention. Early detection and intervention enhance the likelihood of successful treatment and improved outcomes for individuals affected by prostate cancer. Regular screenings and discussions with healthcare providers are essential for maintaining urological health, particularly in the presence of urinary symptoms suggestive of prostate cancer.

4.3.2 Diagnostic Considerations

Presence of blood in urine or semen, when accompanied by other symptoms like changes in urinary patterns or pelvic pain, may raise suspicion for prostate cancer. A thorough examination, including imaging studies and potentially a prostate biopsy, is essential to determine the cause of hematospermia. Prostate cancer may be investigated, particularly if other symptoms or risk factors are identified. Individuals experiencing blood in urine or semen should seek prompt medical attention. Comprehensive evaluation, including imaging studies, blood tests, and potentially a prostate biopsy, is essential for accurate diagnosis and appropriate management.

4.4 Pain Management Strategies:

Multidisciplinary Approach: Addressing pain in advanced prostate cancer requires a multidisciplinary approach involving oncologists, pain specialists, and palliative care teams.

- **Pharmacological Interventions:** Medications, including analgesics and opioids, may be prescribed to manage pain effectively.

- **Interventional Procedures:** Interventional procedures, such as nerve blocks or radiation therapy, may be employed to target specific pain sources.

- **Emotional Impact and Psychosocial Support:** Chronic pain can have emotional repercussions, impacting an individual's mental health and well-being. Psychosocial support is crucial in addressing the holistic impact of pain.

- **End-of-Life Care Considerations: Palliative Care:**
  In cases of advanced prostate cancer with significant pain, palliative care may play a crucial role in enhancing comfort and providing support.

- **Emotional Considerations:** The presence of blood in urine or semen can evoke emotional distress in individuals, underscoring the importance of compassionate communication and support during the diagnostic process.

4.5 Symptoms of Advanced Disease

Pain or discomfort in the pelvic area, lower back, or during ejaculation may occur in advanced stages of prostate cancer, indicating the potential involvement of adjacent structures and tissues. Understanding the nuances of these symptoms is crucial for timely diagnosis, effective management, and enhanced quality of life for individuals affected by advanced prostate cancer:

- **Pelvic Pain or Discomfort:** Pain or discomfort in the pelvic region is a common symptom in advanced prostate cancer. As prostate cancer progresses, the tumor may invade surrounding tissues, including the pelvic bones and nerves. This infiltration can lead to localized pain or discomfort.
- **Lower Back Pain:** Lower back pain is another common symptom associated with advanced prostate cancer. Metastasis to the

bones, particularly the spine, is a characteristic feature of advanced prostate cancer. Tumor involvement in the spine can cause localized pain in the lower back.

- **Ejaculatory Pain:** Pain or discomfort during ejaculation can be indicative of advanced prostate cancer affecting the seminal vesicles. Seminal vesicles, which produce a significant portion of seminal fluid, may be invaded by the tumor. Discomfort during ejaculation can result from the involvement of these structures.

- **Nerve Compression and Pain:** Prostate cancer metastasizing to the spine can lead to nerve compression, causing pain and discomfort. Tumor growth in the spinal column may compress nerves, resulting in radiating pain. Nerve compression can affect the lower back and extend into the pelvic region.

- **Neurological Symptoms:** Advanced prostate cancer that spreads to the nervous system may cause neurological symptoms such as weakness or numbness in the limbs
- **Bone Metastases and Pain:** Advanced prostate cancer often spreads to bones, leading to bone metastases and associated pain. Cancer cells in the bones disrupt the normal bone architecture, causing pain. Bone metastases are a significant source of pain in advanced prostate cancer.
- **Chronic Pain Syndrome**: Individuals with advanced prostate cancer may develop chronic pain syndrome. Persistent pain can lead to changes in the nervous system, resulting in chronic pain. This syndrome may contribute to a continued perception of pain even after the initial stimulus is no longer present.
- **Jaundice:**

In rare cases where the cancer spreads to the liver, jaundice (yellowing of the skin and eyes) may occur

- **Impact on Daily Activities:** Pain and discomfort can significantly impact an individual's ability to perform daily activities. Reduced mobility and discomfort during routine tasks may affect overall quality of life.
- **Changes in Sexual Function**: Prostate cancer, as well as its treatments, can impact sexual function, leading to erectile dysfunction or changes in libido.
- **Bone Pain and Fractures**: Advanced prostate cancer may spread to the bones, causing bone pain, especially in the hips, spine, and pelvis. This can lead to an increased risk of fractures.
- **Weight Loss and Fatigue:**

Unexplained Weight Loss: Unintentional weight loss without changes in diet or exercise can be a symptom of advanced prostate cancer.

Fatigue: Generalized fatigue, weakness, or a decline in overall energy levels may be associated with advanced disease.

- **Swelling in Legs or Pelvis**
  Swelling: Swelling in the legs or pelvic area may occur if the cancer obstructs the flow of urine or lymphatic drainage.

Pain and discomfort in advanced prostate cancer are complex symptoms influenced by the tumor's infiltration into adjacent structures and distant metastases. Recognizing and addressing these symptoms require a comprehensive approach that considers both physical and emotional well-being. Pain management, multidisciplinary care, and psychosocial support contribute to improving the overall quality of life for individuals navigating advanced stages of prostate cancer. Open communication between healthcare providers, patients, and their support networks is essential in tailoring effective strategies for pain control and holistic care.

Chapter 5

Diagnosing Prostate Cancer

Understanding prostate cancer involves recognizing the significance of early detection and the various factors that contribute to its development. Regular screenings, awareness of symptoms, and prompt medical attention play crucial roles in managing and treating prostate cancer effectively. Diagnosing prostate cancer typically involves a combination of tests:

5.1 Digital Rectal Exam(DRE)

The Digital Rectal Exam (DRE) stands as a fundamental component of prostate cancer diagnosis, offering valuable insights into the condition of the prostate gland. This examination, conducted by a healthcare professional, involves the insertion of a gloved, lubricated finger into the rectum to assess the size, texture, shape, and consistency of the prostate. Here is a thorough exploration of the Digital Rectal Exam in the context of diagnosing prostate cancer:

- **Purpose of DRE in Prostate Cancer Diagnosis:**

Early Detection: DRE serves as an integral part of early detection efforts for prostate cancer, allowing for the identification of abnormalities in the prostate gland.

- **Baseline Assessment:** The exam establishes a baseline assessment of the prostate, enabling healthcare providers to monitor changes over time.

5.1.1 Procedure on how to Perform Digital Rectal Exam (DRE).

- **Patient Positioning:** Typically performed with the patient in a bent-over position or lying on their side, the DRE allows optimal access to the rectum.
- **Gloved and Lubricated Finger:** The healthcare professional wears a lubricated glove, ensuring a smooth and comfortable examination.

- **Prostate Palpation:** The examiner gently inserts a finger into the rectum and palpates the posterior surface of the prostate gland.

5.1.2 Assessment of Prostate Characteristics:

- **Size and Consistency:** The examiner evaluates the size, consistency, and any irregularities in the prostate gland.
- **Presence of Nodules or Abnormalities:** The presence of nodules, hard areas, or irregularities may indicate potential issues, including the presence of tumors.

5.1.3 DRE in Conjunction with Other Diagnostic Measures:

PSA Test: Often performed alongside the Prostate-Specific Antigen (PSA) blood test, DRE contributes to a comprehensive diagnostic approach.

Imaging Studies: DRE may be complemented by imaging studies, such as ultrasound or magnetic resonance imaging (MRI), for a more detailed assessment.

5.1.4 Detection of Indicators for Further Evaluation:

Abnormal Findings: Abnormalities detected during DRE, such as hard nodules or asymmetry, may prompt further investigation to determine the nature of the issue.

- DRE findings, in combination with other diagnostic information, aid in risk stratification and guide subsequent steps in the diagnostic process.
- The interpretation of DRE findings can be subjective and dependent on the examiner's experience and skill.
- DRE may have limited sensitivity, and not all prostate cancers may be palpable through this examination alone.

5.1.5 Patient Comfort and Communication:

- **Open Communication:** Healthcare professionals prioritize open communication to ensure patient comfort and consent throughout the procedure.

- **Explanation and Education:** Patients are often provided with explanations of the procedure beforehand, addressing any concerns and emphasizing its importance in prostate health.

5.1.6 Follow-Up and Decision-Making:

- **Informed Decision:** Engage in shared decision-making with the healthcare provider. Discuss the potential benefits and limitations of PSA testing, considering the individual's overall health and preferences.
- **Biopsy Consideration:** Abnormal DRE findings may lead to discussions about the potential need for a prostate biopsy to confirm or rule out cancer.

- **Treatment Planning:** DRE results, in conjunction with other diagnostic information, contribute to treatment planning and decisions regarding the management of prostate cancer.

5.1.7 Continued Advances in Diagnosis:
- **Technological Advancements:** Ongoing advancements, such as the integration of imaging technologies, aim to enhance the accuracy and reliability of prostate cancer diagnosis.
- **Research Contributions:** Ongoing research explores novel methods and technologies to improve the diagnostic capabilities of DRE and enhance its role in early detection.

The Digital Rectal Exam remains an essential tool in the diagnostic arsenal for prostate cancer. Its role in providing valuable clinical information, guiding further diagnostic steps, and contributing to informed decision-making underscores its significance in prostate health. As healthcare practices evolve and technology continues to advance, the integration of DRE with complementary diagnostic approaches promises to enhance the accuracy and efficacy of prostate cancer diagnosis, ultimately benefiting individuals through early detection and improved treatment outcomes.

5.2 Prostate-Specific Antigen (PSA) Test

The Prostate-Specific Antigen (PSA) test is a key tool in the diagnosis and monitoring of prostate

cancer. It measures the levels of a protein produced by the prostate gland in the blood. While widely used, the PSA test is not without controversy and requires careful interpretation. For low-risk prostate cancer cases, PSA tests are often part of active surveillance strategies to monitor progression without immediate intervention. Here's an extensive overview of the PSA test in the context of prostate cancer diagnosis:

5.2.1 Purpose of the PSA Test:
- **Early Detection:** The primary goal of the PSA test is the early detection of prostate cancer. Elevated PSA levels can indicate the presence of abnormal prostate cells.
- **Monitoring:** For individuals with diagnosed prostate cancer, the PSA test is used to monitor the effectiveness of treatment and track disease progression.

5.2.2. Normal PSA Levels:
- **Age-Adjusted Ranges:** Normal PSA levels vary with age, and the test is often interpreted in the context of age-adjusted reference ranges.

- **Baseline PSA:** Establishing a baseline PSA level in younger individuals helps in identifying significant changes over time.

5.2.3. Factors Influencing PSA Levels:

- **Age:** PSA levels tend to increase with age, and this must be considered when evaluating results.
- **Prostate Size:** Enlarged prostates, which can be caused by conditions like benign prostatic hyperplasia (BPH), can elevate PSA levels.
- **Infection or Inflammation:** Prostate infections or inflammation can cause temporary increases in PSA levels.
- **Recent Ejaculation:** Recent sexual activity or ejaculation may transiently elevate PSA levels.

5.2.4. Interpreting PSA Results:

- **Normal Range:** PSA levels within the normal range do not necessarily rule out the presence of prostate cancer. Understand the normal range for PSA levels. Generally, levels below 4 nanograms per milliliter (ng/mL) are considered normal, but age and individual factors are also considered
- **Elevated PSA:** An elevated PSA level may prompt further investigation, such as additional tests or a prostate biopsy, to determine the cause. Elevated PSA level can indicate conditions such as prostate cancer or benign prostatic hyperplasia (BPH).
- **Rate of Change:** The rate of change in PSA levels over time (PSA velocity) can be informative, with a rapid increase potentially raising concern.
- **PSA Velocity and Doubling Time**: The rate at which PSA levels change over time is known as PSA velocity and can be considered in risk assessment.

The time it takes for PSA levels to double is another factor that may influence decision-making in diagnosis and management.

5.2.5 PSA Density:
Adjusting for Prostate Size:
- PSA density (PSA concentration relative to prostate volume). PSA density adjusts PSA levels based on prostate size, helping account for variations related to gland volume.
- An elevated PSA level may lead to a prostate biopsy for a definitive diagnosis. Not all cases of elevated PSA result in a prostate cancer diagnosis.
- If cancer is detected, a Gleason score is assigned based on the aggressiveness of the cancer cells.
- PSA screening is not without controversy due to the risk of false positives and overdiagnosis. Shared decision-making is

essential in determining the appropriateness of screening for an individual.

5.2.6 Advancements and Future Directions

- **Novel Biomarkers:** Ongoing research explores new biomarkers and technologies to enhance the specificity and sensitivity of prostate cancer detection.
- **MRI and Fusion Biopsy:** Multiparametric magnetic resonance imaging (MRI) combined with targeted biopsy (fusion biopsy) is emerging as a complementary diagnostic approach.
- **Exploring Advanced Methods:** Ongoing research explores advanced PSA testing methods, such as measuring specific PSA isoforms, to enhance accuracy and refine risk assessment.

The PSA test remains a valuable tool in the diagnosis and management of prostate cancer, but its interpretation requires careful consideration of various factors. Informed decision-making, personalized risk assessment, and ongoing advancements in diagnostic techniques contribute to the evolving landscape of prostate cancer diagnosis. Regular discussions with healthcare professionals, especially for individuals at higher risk, are essential to navigate the complexities of PSA testing and its implications for prostate health.

5.2.7 Procedure For Estimating Prostate-Specific Antigen (PSA)

levels is a crucial aspect of diagnosing prostate cancer. The PSA test measures the concentration of this protein in the blood, and variations in levels can indicate potential issues with the prostate, including cancer. Here's an overview of the steps involved in estimating PSA for the diagnosis of prostate cancer:

Step 1: Consultation with Healthcare Provider

Begin by consulting with a healthcare provider, especially if there are risk factors such as age, family history, or symptoms that warrant investigation.

Step 2: Baseline PSA Measurement:
Establish a baseline PSA level through a blood test. This initial measurement provides a reference point for future comparisons.

Step 3: Follow-Up Testing:
Depending on the baseline result and individual risk factors, follow-up PSA testing may be scheduled at regular intervals.

Step 4: Confirmatory Procedures: If PSA levels are elevated, a prostate biopsy may be recommended to confirm or rule out prostate cancer.

Step 5: Assessment of Risk: Integrating PSA data with other risk factors, such as Gleason score and imaging results, helps stratify individuals into different risk categories.

Step 6: Monitoring After Treatment: After treatment for prostate cancer, regular PSA testing is often conducted to monitor for any signs of recurrence.

Estimating PSA levels involves a comprehensive approach that considers baseline measurements, risk factors, and ongoing monitoring. It is crucial for individuals to collaborate with healthcare providers, actively participate in decision-making, and undergo additional investigations if needed to confirm or rule out prostate cancer. Regular follow-ups and open communication with healthcare professionals contribute to a more informed and personalized approach to prostate cancer diagnosis and management.

5.3 Prostate Biopsy Procedure

A prostate biopsy is a key diagnostic procedure used to confirm the presence of prostate cancer. If other tests suggest the possibility of cancer, a biopsy is performed, involving the removal of small tissue samples for examination under a microscope.

Types of Prostate Biopsies:

Transrectal Ultrasound (TRUS) Biopsy: This is the most common biopsy method, involving the insertion of a thin needle through the rectum guided by ultrasound imaging.

Transperineal Biopsy: In this approach, the needle is inserted through the perineum, the area between the anus and the scrotum

Prostate biopsy is a diagnostic procedure performed by urologists to obtain tissue samples from the prostate gland for pathological analysis. This comprehensive exploration delves into the intricacies of the prostate biopsy procedure, covering its indications, preparation, execution, and post-procedural considerations

5.3.1 Indications for Prostate Biopsy:

A urologist may recommend a prostate biopsy when there are concerning factors, such as elevated PSA levels, abnormal digital rectal examination (DRE) findings, or suspicion of prostate cancer based on imaging studies. The decision is often made following a thorough assessment of the patient's clinical history and risk factors.

Elevated PSA Levels: A common reason for a prostate biopsy is an elevated Prostate-Specific Antigen (PSA) level, which may indicate prostate abnormalities.

Abnormal Digital Rectal Exam (DRE): If a Digital Rectal Exam (DRE) reveals abnormal findings, it may prompt further investigation through a biopsy.

Monitoring Active Surveillance:
For individuals on active surveillance, periodic biopsies may be performed to monitor changes in the prostate.

5.3.2 Preparation for Prostate Biopsies

Before the biopsy, the urologist discusses the procedure with the patient, explaining the potential risks and benefits. Patients may be advised to discontinue blood-thinning medications and undergo an enema to ensure the rectum is clear for a more accurate biopsy.

Patient Education and Support: Education and counseling are crucial components, ensuring individuals are well-informed about the biopsy process, potential outcomes, and available support.

Shared Decision-Making: The decision to undergo a prostate biopsy involves shared decision-making between the patient and healthcare provider, considering individual health status and preferences.

5.3.3 Prostate Biopsies Execution

Anesthesia and Antibiotic Administration

Before the biopsy, the urologist administers a local anesthetic to the prostate, typically in the form of a numbing medication. This minimizes discomfort during the procedure. In addition, a short course of antibiotics may be prescribed to reduce the risk of infection.

Transrectal Ultrasound (TRUS) Guidance:

TRUS is commonly employed to guide the biopsy procedure. It involves the insertion of a lubricated ultrasound probe into the rectum, providing real-time imaging of the prostate. The urologist uses this visual guidance to target specific areas for biopsy. During a TRUS biopsy, the ultrasound helps guide the needle to specific areas of the prostate for tissue sampling.

Biopsy Needle Insertion: A thin biopsy needle is then inserted through the ultrasound probe, reaching the prostate gland. The urologist carefully maneuvers the needle to obtain multiple tissue samples from different areas of the prostate

Sampling Multiple Cores: Multiple tissue samples, or cores, are typically collected from different regions of the prostate to increase diagnostic accuracy. The urologist often employs a multiple core biopsy technique, obtaining samples from various regions of the prostate. This approach improves the chances of detecting cancerous tissue and provides a more comprehensive assessment.

Specimen Collection:

Each tissue sample, known as a core, is collected and labeled for subsequent analysis by a pathologist. The pathologist examines the samples under a microscope to determine the presence and characteristics of cancer cells.

Recommendations for Further Testing:

Imaging Studies: In cases where biopsy results are inconclusive or further details are needed, additional imaging studies, such as multiparametric MRI, may be recommended.

Repeat Biopsy:

If initial biopsy results are ambiguous, inconclusive, or if there are persistent concerns, a repeat biopsy may be suggested

5.3.4 Post-Biopsy Considerations:

Pathology Evaluation: Tissue samples are sent to a pathology lab where they are examined under a microscope to determine if cancer cells are present.

Gleason Score:

The Gleason score, a grading system for prostate cancer, is derived from the biopsy results and helps assess the cancer's aggressiveness.

Discussing Results:

Healthcare providers discuss biopsy results with patients, providing information about the cancer's stage and treatment options.

Post-Biopsy Care:

After the procedure, patients are monitored for a short period to ensure there are no immediate complications. They are given instructions for post-biopsy care, which may include guidelines on activities, medications, and the monitoring of any potential side effects.

5.3.5. Potential Side Effects of Prostate Biopsy Procedure

While generally considered safe, the prostate biopsy procedure may result in temporary side effects. These can include minor bleeding, discomfort, or a small risk of infection. Patients are advised to report any unusual symptoms to their urologist promptly

Infection:

Infection is a potential risk, and individuals are monitored for signs of infection post-biopsy.

Bleeding:

Some bleeding may occur, leading to blood in the urine or semen, but it's usually temporary.

Pain and Discomfort:

Pain and discomfort are common but can be managed with medications.

5.3.6. Pathological Analysis and Follow-Up:

The collected tissue samples undergo thorough pathological analysis. The results are shared with the patient, guiding further management decisions. Depending on the findings, the urologist discusses appropriate follow-up, potential treatment options, or the need for addiConclusion:

The prostate biopsy procedure, conducted by a skilled urologist, is a pivotal step in the diagnostic journey for prostate-related concerns. From meticulous preparation and guidance using TRUS to the collection of tissue samples and post-biopsy care, the procedure is orchestrated to ensure accurate results and patient comfort. Continuous advancements in technology and techniques contribute to the refinement of prostate biopsy procedures, enhancing diagnostic accuracy and patient outcomes

5.3.7. Interpreting Biopsy Results

Prostate biopsy results are integral to confirming or ruling out prostate cancer and guiding subsequent treatment decisions. This comprehensive exploration delves into the diverse outcomes that can emerge from a prostate biopsy, detailing the various aspects of interpretation and the implications for individuals undergoing this diagnostic procedure.

Interpretation with Gleason Score and Grading:
Gleason Score: A crucial component of biopsy results is the Gleason score, which assesses the

aggressiveness of prostate cancer based on tissue architecture. Scores typically range from 6 to 10.

Gleason Grading:

Biopsy results may include a Gleason grade, reflecting how closely the cancerous tissue resembles normal prostate tissue. Higher grades indicate more aggressive cancers.

1. Normal/Benign Results:

Absence of Cancer Cells: A normal or benign biopsy result indicates the absence of cancer cells in the sampled prostate tissue.

The tissue samples may reveal typical, non-cancerous components of the prostate, such as glandular structures and stroma.

2. Atypical or Suspicious Result

Atypical Small Acinar Proliferation (ASAP):

- This result suggests abnormal cellular growth that falls short of a definitive cancer diagnosis but warrants close monitoring and potential further investigation.

High-Grade Prostatic Intraepithelial Neoplasia (PIN):
PIN indicates abnormal cell changes in the prostate that may be associated with an increased risk of developing prostate cancer.

5.3.8 Cancer Detection:
Presence of Cancer Cells: Positive biopsy results confirm the presence of cancer cells within the sampled prostate tissue.

Cancer Location and Size:
The biopsy provides information about the location and extent of cancer within the prostate, aiding in staging.

Staging Information:
Tumor Stage: Biopsy results contribute to determining the tumor stage, which indicates the

extent of cancer within the prostate and whether it has spread beyond.

Lymph Node Involvement:
Information on lymph node involvement is crucial for understanding the potential spread of cancer.

Multifocality:
Multifocal Cancer: Biopsies may reveal multifocal cancer, indicating the presence of cancer in multiple regions of the prostate.

5.3.9 Advancements in Biopsy Techniques:
Multiparametric MRI Fusion Biopsy: Advanced imaging techniques, such as multiparametric MRI fusion biopsy, combine MRI images with real-time ultrasound guidance for more precise targeting.

Liquid Biopsy: Emerging technologies, like liquid biopsies, are being explored to detect circulating tumor DNA in the blood.

5.3.10 Post-Treatment Monitoring:

Treatment Decision-Making:

Informed Treatment Choices: Biopsy results play a pivotal role in guiding treatment decisions, helping individuals and healthcare providers choose appropriate interventions based on the cancer's characteristics.

Monitoring Recurrence: For individuals who undergo treatment, biopsy results may influence post-treatment monitoring strategies to detect any signs of recurrence.

Patient Counseling:

Discussing Results with Patients: Healthcare providers engage in detailed discussions with patients to explain biopsy results, discuss potential treatment options, and address any concerns.

Interpreting prostate biopsy results involves a nuanced analysis of cellular characteristics, staging information, and the Gleason score, all of which collectively guide treatment decisions. Patient counseling, thorough discussions with healthcare providers, and ongoing support are crucial components of the diagnostic process, ensuring individuals receive comprehensive information to make informed choices in the management of prostate cancer.

Chapter 6

Importance of Early Detection in Prostate Cancer

The Importance of Early Detection in Prostate Cancer: Early detection is a cornerstone in the battle against prostate cancer, as it significantly influences treatment outcomes, quality of life, and the overall prognosis for individuals diagnosed with the disease. Understanding the importance of early detection involves recognizing the potential benefits and the various methods available for screening and diagnosis. Raising awareness about the importance of early detection through educational campaigns encourages regular screenings and informed decision-making.

Screening Methods for Early Detection:

1. PSA Test:

Regular prostate-specific antigen (PSA) testing is a common method for early detection. Elevated PSA levels may indicate the presence of prostate cancer or other prostate conditions, prompting further investigation.

2. Digital Rectal Exam (DRE):

Physical examination of the prostate through the rectum helps assess its size, texture, and the presence of any abnormalities.

3. Imaging Studies:

Advanced imaging techniques, such as magnetic resonance imaging (MRI), may assist in identifying suspicious areas within the prostate.

6.1 Increased Treatment Options

Prostate Cancer show silent progression from asymptomatic at early Stages to serious complications if the necessary intervention is not administered. Prostate cancer often progresses silently in its early stages, exhibiting minimal to no symptoms. This makes routine screening vital for timely detection. Early detection allows for a broader range of treatment options. When prostate cancer is diagnosed in its early stages, treatment interventions like surgery, radiation therapy, and active surveillance are more viable. These options are often associated with higher success rates and fewer side effects.

Early detection brings Improved Prognosis and enhanced survival rates. Identifying prostate cancer at an early stage allows for a more favorable prognosis. Early intervention increases the likelihood of successful treatment and long-term remission. Early-stage prostate cancer is associated with higher survival rates. Treatment interventions are often more effective when the cancer is localized.

6.2 Preserving Quality of Life

Early intervention can contribute to preserving normal urinary and sexual function. Treatment options for localized prostate cancer, such as nerve-sparing surgery or targeted radiation therapy, aim to minimize the impact on these critical aspects of a man's quality of life. Early detection of prostate cancer plays a pivotal role in preserving the quality of life for individuals facing this diagnosis. This comprehensive exploration delves into the various aspects through which early detection contributes to maintaining a higher quality of life, considering both the physical and emotional dimensions.

6.2.1. Maintaining Normal Activities and Sexual Functions: With early detection, treatment interventions are more targeted and may allow individuals to maintain their normal daily activities. This includes work, social engagements, and physical activities, contributing to a sense of normalcy.

Less invasive treatments for early-stage prostate cancer aim to preserve sexual function. This is crucial for maintaining intimate relationships and supporting emotional well-being.
.

6.2.2. Avoiding Advanced Disease Complications: Early detection prevents the progression of prostate cancer to advanced stages, where complications and symptoms are more severe. This avoidance of advanced disease contributes to a better overall quality of life.

Early detection allows for a range of treatment options, often less aggressive than those required for advanced-stage cancer. This minimizes potential side effects such as incontinence and erectile dysfunction, which can significantly impact the overall quality of life.

6.2.3. Enhancing Treatment Success Rates: Treating prostate cancer at an early stage increases the likelihood of treatment success. Successful treatment not only addresses the physical aspects of the disease but also positively influences emotional and mental well-being. For certain low-risk cases, early detection enables active surveillance rather than immediate aggressive treatment. This approach minimizes treatment-related side effects, allowing individuals to maintain a relatively normal life.

6.2.4 Improving Emotional Well-Being: Knowing that prostate cancer is detected early provides individuals with a sense of control over their health. This knowledge contributes to improved emotional well-being, reducing anxiety and fear associated with a more advanced disease. A diagnosis of cancer can have significant psychological implications. Early detection provides individuals with more treatment choices and a potentially less daunting journey, reducing the psychological burden associated with aggressive treatments

6.2.5. Empowering Informed Decision-Making: Early detection empowers individuals to actively participate in their healthcare decisions. Informed decision-making allows for choices that align with personal preferences, values, and the desire for a balanced quality of life. For certain low-risk cases, early detection enables active surveillance rather than immediate aggressive treatment. This approach minimizes treatment-related side effects, allowing individuals to maintain a relatively normal life.

6.2.6 Supporting Long-Term Quality of Life: By addressing prostate cancer at an early stage, the overall impact on the individual's life is more manageable. This contributes to long-term well-being, allowing individuals to continue to enjoy a fulfilling and meaningful life. Preserving the quality of life through early detection of prostate cancer goes beyond medical interventions. It encompasses a holistic approach that considers physical health, emotional well-being, and individual choices. Early detection provides a pathway to a more balanced and fulfilling life, enabling individuals to navigate the complexities of a prostate cancer diagnosis with resilience and optimism.

6.3 Improving Prognosis

Early detection of prostate cancer is a linchpin in enhancing the prognosis for individuals facing this diagnosis. This in-depth exploration delves into the multifaceted ways in which early detection contributes to improved prognoses, covering aspects from treatment effectiveness to long-term survival rates.

6.3.1. Increased Treatment Options: Early detection broadens the spectrum of treatment options available. This diversity allows healthcare providers to tailor interventions based on the individual's health status, preferences, and the specific characteristics of the cancer, optimizing the chances of successful treatment. Detecting prostate cancer at an early stage often allows for localized treatment interventions. These may include surgery, radiation therapy, or focal therapies that specifically target the cancerous cells within the prostate, leading to more effective treatment.

6.3.2. Curative Intent: Prostate cancer diagnosed early is often approached with curative intent. This means that the goal of treatment is not just to manage the symptoms but to eliminate the cancer entirely, leading to a more positive prognosis. Early-stage prostate cancer is associated with higher survival rates. Treatment interventions at this stage are often more successful, contributing to extended life expectancy and improved overall outcomes.

6.3.3 Reduced Risk of Metastasis: Detecting and treating prostate cancer early significantly reduces the risk of metastasis, the spread of cancer to other parts of the body. This pivotal factor contributes to a more favorable prognosis, as localized cancer is generally more manageable. Early detection allows for risk-adapted approaches, tailoring the intensity of treatment to the specific characteristics of the cancer. This personalized strategy optimizes outcomes and minimizes unnecessary interventions for low-risk cases.

6.3.4 Precise Staging Information: Early detection provides precise staging information, indicating the extent of cancer within the prostate and whether it has spread to surrounding tissues or lymph nodes. This information guides treatment planning and contributes to a more accurate prognosis. Early detection facilitates the determination of the Gleason score, a crucial factor in assessing the aggressiveness of the cancer. This risk stratification guides treatment decisions, ensuring a personalized approach to managing the disease.

6.3.5 Quality of Life Considerations: Early detection considers not only the physical aspects of treatment but also the individual's overall quality of life. This holistic approach supports emotional and psychological well-being, further enhancing the overall prognosis After successful treatment, individuals with early-detected prostate cancer undergo post-treatment monitoring. This vigilant approach ensures that any signs of recurrence are promptly addressed, further contributing to a positive prognosis.

Early detection of prostate cancer is pivotal in transforming the landscape of prognosis. It not only increases the effectiveness of treatment but also shapes a comprehensive and personalized approach to managing the disease. From localized interventions to enhanced survival rates, the benefits of early detection ripple through various facets, ultimately contributing to a more positive prognosis for individuals facing prostate cancer.

6.4 Reversing Prostate Cancer at Early Detection: An In-Depth Exploration

While it's crucial to emphasize that the idea of "reversing" prostate cancer requires careful consideration, early detection opens avenues for effective management and treatment that can significantly improve outcomes. This comprehensive exploration delves into the multifaceted steps and interventions that can be taken to address prostate cancer detected at an early stage.

6.4.1. Multidisciplinary Consultation: Upon early detection, a multidisciplinary approach is crucial. Consultation with a team of healthcare professionals, including urologists, oncologists, and radiation oncologists, ensures a comprehensive understanding of the individual case. Precise risk assessment, including factors such as the Gleason score, PSA levels, and imaging studies, helps stratify the risk associated with the cancer. This guides decision-making regarding the intensity and type of treatment.

6.4.2. Treatment Options: Early detection offers a range of treatment options, including surgery, radiation therapy, hormone therapy, and active surveillance. Tailoring the treatment approach to the specific characteristics of the cancer optimizes the chances of success. For cases with lower risk, active surveillance may be a viable option. This involves close monitoring through regular check-ups, PSA tests, and periodic imaging to assess any changes in the cancer's behavior.

6.4.3. Surgery and Radiation Therapy: Prostatectomy, the surgical removal of the prostate gland, may be recommended for localized cancers. Advances in surgical techniques, such as robotic-assisted surgery, contribute to reduced recovery times and improved outcomes.

Various forms of radiation therapy, including external beam radiation and brachytherapy, target cancer cells with precision. This helps eliminate or shrink the tumor while minimizing damage to surrounding healthy tissue.

6.4.4. Hormone Therapy: Hormone therapy aims to suppress the activity of hormones like testosterone, which fuel the growth of some prostate cancers. It may be used alone or in combination with other treatments, particularly for more advanced cases.

6.4.5 Advanced Imaging Techniques: Advanced imaging, such as multiparametric MRI, aids in precise tumor localization and staging. This information guides treatment decisions and contributes to a more effective intervention strategy.

6.4.6 Nutritional and Lifestyle Interventions: Adopting a healthy lifestyle, including a balanced diet rich in antioxidants, regular exercise, and stress management, may support overall well-being. While not a standalone treatment, these interventions contribute to a holistic approach to health.

6.4.7. Clinical Trials and Emerging Therapies: Participation in clinical trials and exploring emerging therapies can be considered. These avenues may offer innovative treatments and contribute to advancing the understanding of prostate cancer management.

6.4.8. Supportive Care and Emotional Well-Being: Addressing the emotional and psychological aspects of a prostate cancer diagnosis is vital. Supportive care, including counseling and involvement in support groups, contributes to a holistic approach to health and well-being.

6.4.9. Post-Treatment Monitoring: Regular post-treatment monitoring, involving PSA tests, imaging studies, and check-ups, ensures the ongoing assessment of treatment effectiveness and the detection of any signs of recurrence.

Addressing prostate cancer detected at an early stage involves a multifaceted and individualized approach. From treatment options to lifestyle interventions and emotional support, these steps collectively contribute to managing and, in many cases, effectively addressing the disease. The collaboration between healthcare professionals and individuals facing prostate cancer is essential in navigating the complexities of treatment and striving for positive outcomes.

6.5 Other Benefits of Prostate Cancer Early detection

Shared Decision-Making: The decision to undergo screening involves shared decision-making between individuals and healthcare providers, considering factors like age, health status, and preferences. Patient are Empowered for Informed Decision-Making. Early detection empowers individuals to make informed decisions about their health, fostering a proactive approach to managing their well-being.

Risk Stratification: Early detection allows for the identification of individuals at higher risk, such as those with a family history or specific risk factors, enabling tailored screening strategies.

Global Impact on Cancer Burden: A focus on early detection contributes to reducing the global burden of prostate cancer. Addressing cases at an earlier, more manageable stage not only saves lives on an individual level but also has a positive impact on a broader scale

Improved Survival Rates: The correlation between early detection and improved survival rates is well-established. Prostate cancer, when identified at an early, localized stage, has a high likelihood of successful treatment and long-term survival. Timely intervention can prevent the cancer from advancing to a more aggressive and challenging-to-treat stage.

Early detection enables the identification of individuals at higher risk, such as those with a family history or specific risk factors. Tailored screening strategies can be implemented for this group, enhancing precision in diagnosis.

Early detection of Prostate Cancer leads to Proactive Health Management. Early detection fosters a proactive approach to managing prostate health. Regular screenings and check-ups become a routine part of healthcare, contributing to overall well-being and preventive care.

Reduced Treatment Intensity: Detecting prostate cancer early may allow for less aggressive treatment approaches, minimizing potential side effects and preserving a higher quality of life. In some cases, especially with slow-growing tumors, active surveillance might be a suitable option, avoiding unnecessary interventions and minimizing the impact on a person's quality of life.

Minimized Spread and Metastasis: Early detection helps prevent the spread of cancer beyond the prostate. Prostate cancer, when confined to the prostate gland, is more manageable and often curable. Once it metastasizes to other organs, the complexity of treatment increases, and the chances of cure decrease. Detecting and treating prostate cancer early reduces the risk of metastasis, preventing the spread of cancer to other organs.

Cost-Effectiveness: From a healthcare system perspective, early detection is often more cost-effective. Treating prostate cancer in its early stages requires less intensive and costly interventions compared to managing advanced-stage cancer, which may involve prolonged and resource-intensive treatments.

Psychological Well-being: Early detection can alleviate anxiety and uncertainty associated with an undiagnosed or untreated condition. Knowing the status of one's health allows individuals and their families to make informed decisions, plan for the future, and engage in supportive care measures.

Community Health Impact: A focus on early detection contributes to public health efforts by reducing the overall burden of advanced-stage prostate cancer. Regular screening and awareness campaigns can lead to earlier diagnoses on a broader scale, positively impacting community health.

early detection is a crucial factor in effectively managing prostate cancer. Through regular screenings and awareness, individuals can take proactive steps toward preserving their health, accessing a wider range of treatment options, and ultimately improving their chances of a positive outcome in the face of prostate cancer.

CHAPTER 7

Further Screening and Testing for Prostate Cancer

Screening and testing for prostate cancer typically involve a combination of methods aimed at detecting the presence of cancer or assessing the risk of its development. It's important to note that the decision to undergo screening should be based on informed discussions between individuals and their healthcare providers, taking into account individual risk factors and preferences. Common screening methods include:

Underlying Principle For Prostate Diagnostic Procedure

A) **Prostate-Specific Antigen (PSA) Test:**

What It Measures: PSA is a protein produced by the prostate gland. Elevated levels may indicate the presence of prostate cancer, but other factors can also influence PSA levels.

How It's Done: A blood sample is taken and analyzed for PSA levels.

Considerations: High PSA levels do not definitively diagnose cancer but may prompt further investigation.

B) Digital Rectal Exam (DRE):

What It Involves: A physical examination where a healthcare provider inserts a gloved, lubricated finger into the rectum to feel the prostate for abnormalities.

Purpose: DRE helps assess the size, texture, and presence of lumps or irregularities in the prostate.

Considerations: DRE is often performed in conjunction with the PSA test for a more comprehensive evaluation.

C) Multiparametric Magnetic Resonance Imaging (mpMRI):

What It Involves: Advanced imaging technique using MRI to create detailed images of the prostate.

Purpose: Helps identify suspicious areas that may require further investigation, such as biopsy.

Considerations: mpMRI is increasingly used for targeted biopsies, improving the accuracy of cancer detection.

D) . Genetic Testing:

What It Involves: Analyzing genes associated with an increased risk of prostate cancer, such as BRCA1 and BRCA2.

Purpose: Identifies individuals with a higher genetic predisposition, influencing screening frequency and potential preventive measures.

Considerations: Genetic testing may be recommended for those with a family history of prostate cancer.

E). Nomograms and Risk Calculators:

What They Are: Tools that estimate an individual's risk of having prostate cancer based on various factors, including age, family history, and PSA levels.

Purpose: Assists in decision-making regarding further diagnostic tests or surveillance.

Considerations: Nomograms provide a personalized risk assessment.

It's crucial for individuals to discuss the potential benefits and risks of screening with their healthcare providers, considering factors such as age, overall health, family history, and personal preferences. Informed decision-making is key to optimizing the effectiveness of prostate cancer screening and testing.

7.1 An In-Depth Exploration of Prostate Health Index (phi)

The Prostate Health Index (phi) has emerged as a valuable tool in the diagnosis and management of prostate cancer. This comprehensive exploration delves into the intricacies of phi, its components, and its role in providing more accurate information for healthcare professionals in assessing the risk of prostate cancer. The Prostate Health Index, abbreviated as phi, is a blood test that combines multiple prostate-specific markers to provide a more nuanced assessment of prostate health compared to traditional methods like the PSA (Prostate-Specific Antigen) test.

7.1.1 Prostate Health Index (phi) Procedure

What It Measures: A combination of PSA, free PSA, and p2PSA. It provides a more specific risk assessment than PSA alone.

How It's Done: Blood test similar to the PSA test.

Considerations: phi may offer additional information to better distinguish between benign conditions and prostate cancer.

Components of Prostate Health Index:

The phi test incorporates three main components:

PSA: Measures the total amount of PSA in the blood.

Free PSA: Assesses the percentage of PSA not bound to proteins.

p2PSA: Evaluates a specific form of free PSA associated with prostate cancer.

Importance of Prostate Health Index (Phi):
- Enhanced Specificity for Prostate Cancer Detection:
- Phi Risk Stratification
- Reduction of Unnecessary Biopsies
- Clinical Validity and Guidelines:
- Combining phi with Imaging Studies Enhances Detection of Prostate Cancer
- Monitoring Prostate Cancer Patients

Enhanced Specificity for Prostate Cancer Detection:

The combination of PSA, free PSA, and p2PSA in phi offers enhanced specificity, providing a more refined evaluation of the likelihood of prostate cancer. This can help differentiate between benign conditions and potential malignancies.

Phi Risk Stratification

Phi contributes to a more precise risk stratification, assisting healthcare professionals in categorizing individuals into different risk groups. This aids in personalized decision-making regarding further diagnostic tests and potential treatment strategies.

Reduction of Unnecessary Biopsies:

By improving specificity, phi helps reduce the number of unnecessary prostate biopsies. This is particularly valuable in preventing overdiagnosis and overtreatment, aligning with the principles of personalized medicine.

Clinical Validity and Guidelines:
Phi has demonstrated clinical validity, and its incorporation into clinical guidelines reflects its growing importance in prostate cancer diagnosis. It complements existing tools and provides additional information for a comprehensive assessment.

Enhances Accuracy of Detection and Localization
Integrating phi with advanced imaging studies, such as multiparametric MRI, offers a holistic approach to prostate cancer diagnosis. The combination enhances the accuracy of detection and localization, guiding subsequent interventions.

8. Monitoring Prostate Cancer Patients:
Phi is not limited to initial diagnosis; it also plays a role in monitoring prostate cancer patients. Serial

measurements can provide valuable information on disease progression or response to treatment over time.

7.1.4. Phi Considerations and Limitations:

While phi is a valuable tool, it's essential to consider its limitations. Factors such as age, prostate volume, and certain medical conditions can influence phi results. Healthcare professionals must interpret phi in the context of individual patient characteristics.

7 1.5 Patient Education and Awareness on Phi

Patient education is crucial in promoting awareness of phi and its role in prostate health. Informed patients can engage in shared decision-making with healthcare providers, fostering a proactive approach to their well-being.

The Prostate Health Index (phi) represents a significant advancement in prostate cancer diagnosis, offering a more nuanced and specific evaluation compared to traditional methods. As an integral part of the diagnostic landscape, phi contributes to personalized medicine by reducing unnecessary interventions and enhancing risk stratification. Its integration into clinical guidelines underscores its importance in modern prostate health management.

7.2 Multiparametric Magnetic Resonance Imaging (mpMRI) in Prostate Cancer Detection

Multiparametric Magnetic Resonance Imaging (mpMRI) has revolutionized the landscape of prostate cancer diagnosis, providing a detailed and multi-faceted approach to imaging. This in-depth exploration delves into the intricacies of mpMRI, its components, and its pivotal role in enhancing the accuracy of prostate cancer detection.

mpMRI is a sophisticated imaging technique that combines multiple parameters, including anatomical, functional, and diffusion-weighted imaging, to provide a comprehensive view of the prostate gland.

7.2.1 Components of mpMRI:

The key components of mpMRI include:

T2-weighted Imaging: Offers detailed anatomical information.

Diffusion-weighted Imaging (DWI): Measures the movement of water molecules, aiding in detecting abnormalities.

Dynamic Contrast-Enhanced (DCE) Imaging: Highlights areas with increased blood flow, often indicative of cancerous tissue.

7.2.2 Advantages of mpMRI in Prostate Cancer Detection

Improved Localization and Visualization:
mpMRI enables precise localization of suspicious areas within the prostate, improving the visualization of potential cancerous lesions. This accuracy assists in targeted biopsies and treatment planning.

Risk Stratification:
mpMRI contributes to risk stratification by distinguishing between low-risk and high-risk lesions. This information guides healthcare professionals in determining the appropriate course of action, avoiding unnecessary interventions for indolent cases.

Role in Fusion Biopsy:
Fusion biopsy, combining mpMRI images with real-time ultrasound, enhances the accuracy of prostate biopsies. Targeting suspicious areas identified by mpMRI reduces the likelihood of missing clinically significant cancers.

Reducing Unnecessary Biopsies:

mpMRI's ability to identify lesions with a higher likelihood of being clinically significant helps reduce unnecessary biopsies for low-risk cases. This aligns with the principles of precision medicine and patient-centered care.

Impact on Treatment Decision-Making:

The information derived from mpMRI significantly influences treatment decision-making. It aids in determining the appropriate management strategy, whether through active surveillance, localized interventions, or more aggressive treatments for high-risk cases.

Follow-up and Monitoring:

mpMRI isn't limited to initial diagnosis; it plays a crucial role in follow-up and monitoring. Sequential imaging allows healthcare professionals to track disease progression, assess treatment response, and adapt management strategies accordingly.

Patient Empowerment and Informed Decision-Making:

mpMRI empowers patients by providing clear visualizations and facilitating informed decision-making. Patients actively participating in their healthcare journey can engage in shared decision-making with their healthcare providers.

7.2.3 Considerations and Challenges

While mpMRI is a powerful diagnostic tool, considerations such as operator expertise, equipment quality, and interpretation challenges must be acknowledged. Addressing these aspects ensures optimal utilization of mpMRI in clinical practice.

Multiparametric Magnetic Resonance Imaging (mpMRI) stands at the forefront of prostate cancer diagnosis, offering a comprehensive and precise approach to imaging. Its integration into clinical practice has transformed the landscape of prostate health, providing valuable insights for risk assessment, biopsy guidance, and treatment planning. As technology continues to advance, mpMRI is poised to play an increasingly pivotal role in enhancing the accuracy of prostate cancer detection and improving patient outcomes.

7.3 Genetic Testing for Prostate Cancer:

Genetic testing has become a crucial component in the landscape of prostate cancer diagnosis and risk assessment. This extensive exploration delves into the intricacies of genetic testing, its significance in understanding prostate cancer susceptibility, and its impact on personalized treatment and prevention strategies.

7.3.1. Identifying Hereditary Risk Factors:

Genetic testing for prostate cancer has evolved with advancements in genomic research. It encompasses a range of techniques to identify specific genetic alterations associated with an increased risk of developing prostate cancer.

Genetic testing aims to identify hereditary risk factors linked to prostate cancer. Key genes, such as BRCA1, BRCA2, and HOXB13, are among those associated with an elevated risk. Identifying these genetic markers informs risk assessment and management strategies.

Germline and Somatic Mutations: Genetic testing distinguishes between germline and somatic mutations. Germline mutations are present in every cell of an individual's body and can be inherited, while somatic mutations occur specifically in the prostate cells and are not passed on to offspring.

7.3.2 Purpose of Genetic testing in Prostate Cancer.

- **Risk Stratification and Counseling:** Genetic testing contributes to risk stratification by identifying individuals with an increased genetic predisposition to prostate cancer. Genetic counselors play a crucial role in interpreting results, providing informed counseling, and guiding individuals in making informed decisions based on their genetic risk.

- **Familial and Inherited Patterns:** Understanding familial and inherited patterns is essential. Genetic testing helps identify whether an individual has inherited specific genetic mutations associated with an elevated risk, providing valuable information for both the individual and their family members.

- **Impact on Treatment Decision-Making:** Genetic testing influences treatment decision-making by providing insights into the aggressiveness of prostate cancer. Individuals with certain genetic mutations may benefit from targeted therapies, and their treatment plans can be personalized based on genetic information.

- **Early Detection and Prevention Strategies:** Genetic testing facilitates early detection and prevention strategies. It aids in identifying individuals at higher risk, allowing for more vigilant screening and surveillance. Proactive measures, such as lifestyle modifications or preventive interventions, can be implemented based on genetic risk.

- **Implications for Family Members:** Positive genetic test results have implications for family members. Testing allows at-risk relatives to undergo genetic testing themselves and adopt personalized prevention or surveillance strategies if needed.

7.3.3 Challenges and Ethical Considerations: Challenges, including the interpretation of variants of uncertain significance and the potential psychological impact of genetic information, must be addressed. Ethical considerations, such as privacy and the potential for genetic discrimination, are also crucial aspects of genetic testing.

7.3.4 Future Directions in Precision Medicine: Genetic testing is at the forefront of precision medicine for prostate cancer. Ongoing research explores additional genetic markers, potential therapeutic targets, and the integration of genetic information into broader precision medicine approaches.

Genetic testing for prostate cancer represents a transformative leap in understanding individual susceptibility, guiding treatment decisions, and informing preventive strategies. As technology continues to advance, the integration of genetic information into the realm of prostate cancer care holds promise for more personalized, targeted, and effective approaches to diagnosis, treatment, and prprevention.

7.4 Practical Guide to Prostate Biopsy Procedures.

Biopsy: Involves removal of small tissue samples from the prostate for examination under a microscope.

Purpose: To confirms the presence of cancer, determines its aggressiveness (Gleason score), and guides treatment decisions.

Considerations: Biopsy is often recommended if PSA levels are elevated or if abnormalities are found in imaging studies.

Biopsy is a pivotal procedure in confirming the presence of prostate cancer, providing crucial information about the type, grade, and extent of the disease. Understanding the various biopsy techniques, their significance, and what to expect during and after the procedure is essential for individuals undergoing prostate cancer diagnosis.

7.4.1. Why Biopsy is Necessary:

- **Confirmation of Cancer:** Biopsy is the definitive method for confirming the presence of cancerous cells in the prostate.
- **Determining Grade and Stage:** It helps assess the aggressiveness (Gleason score) and stage of the cancer, crucial for treatment planning.
- **Guiding Treatment Decisions:** Biopsy results guide healthcare providers in recommending appropriate treatment strategies based on the specific characteristics of the cancer.

7.4.2. Types of Prostate Biopsy:

The three types of prostate biopsy are

- Transrectal Ultrasound (TRUS) Biopsy
- Transperineal Biopsy
- MRI-Guided Biopsy

Transrectal Ultrasound (TRUS) Biopsy:

Procedure: A thin, ultrasound probe is inserted into the rectum to visualize the prostate. Guided by ultrasound images, a biopsy needle collects small tissue samples from different areas of the prostate.

Considerations: Commonly used, minimally invasive, and well-tolerated. It may cause some discomfort, and antibiotics are often prescribed to prevent infection.

Transperineal Biopsy:

Procedure: A biopsy needle is inserted through the perineum, the area between the scrotum and anus, to collect tissue samples from the prostate.

Considerations: This approach is used when transrectal biopsy is not feasible or to target specific areas of the prostate.

MRI-Guided Biopsy:

Procedure: Combining Magnetic Resonance Imaging (MRI) with biopsy, this approach allows for targeted sampling of suspicious areas identified on imaging.

Considerations: Enhances precision and accuracy in detecting significant tumors, reducing the likelihood of underdiagnosis.

7.4.3. Preparing for a Prostate Biopsy:

- **Discussion with Healthcare Provider:**

  Importance: Discuss the procedure, potential risks, and benefits with the healthcare provider.

  Informed Consent: Obtain informed consent, understanding the purpose and potential outcomes of the biopsy.

- **Antibiotics:**

  Prevention of Infection: Antibiotics are often prescribed before and after the biopsy to minimize the risk of infection.

- **Bowel Preparation:**

Minimizing Contamination: In the case of a transrectal biopsy, bowel preparation, such as an enema, may be advised to minimize contamination.

7.4.4. During the Biopsy Procedure:

- **Local Anesthesia and Pain Management:** Local anesthesia is administered to numb the area, reducing discomfort during the procedure.

- **Biopsy Needle Placement:**
- **Precision:** The biopsy needle is carefully guided into the prostate to collect small tissue samples.
- **Multiple Samples Collection**
- **Comprehensive Assessment:** Multiple samples are typically collected from different areas of the prostate to ensure a comprehensive assessment.

7.4.5. After the Biopsy:

- **Recovery Period:** Most individuals can resume normal activities shortly after the procedure.
- **Possible Discomfort:** Some may experience minor discomfort or blood in the urine or semen, which usually resolves within a few days.
- **Pathology Analysis:** Tissue samples are sent to a pathologist for analysis, providing a definitive diagnosis and details about the cancer's characteristics.
- **Follow-up Discussions:** Follow-up discussions with the healthcare provider involve understanding biopsy results and discussing further steps, including treatment options.

Understanding the significance of biopsy procedures in prostate cancer diagnosis empowers individuals to actively participate in their healthcare journey. Open communication with healthcare providers, adherence to pre-biopsy preparations, and post-biopsy follow-up contribute to a comprehensive and informed approach to prostate cancer diagnosis and subsequent treatment planning.

CHAPTER 8

Classification of Prostate Cancer (1)

Categorizing Prostate Cancer: An In-Depth Exploration

Categorizing prostate cancer involves a comprehensive assessment of various factors to determine the extent, aggressiveness, and appropriate management strategies. This extensive exploration delves into the intricate process of categorizing prostate cancer, including staging, grading, and risk stratification. Staging and grading systems offer a comprehensive framework for classifying and understanding prostate cancer. Staging assesses the extent of cancer spread, while grading evaluates the cancer's aggressiveness.

8.1. Introduction to Staging and Grading:

Staging Prostate Cancer: Staging assesses the extent of prostate cancer, determining if and how far the cancer has spread beyond the prostate. The TNM system (Tumor, Nodes, Metastasis) is commonly used, providing a standardized framework for categorizing the disease based on tumor size, lymph node involvement, and metastasis

8.1.1 TNM Staging System:

Tumor (T): Describes the primary tumor's size and extent. Ranges from T1 (confined to the prostate) to T4 (spread to adjacent structures).

Node (N): Evaluates whether cancer has spread to nearby lymph nodes. N0 indicates no lymph node involvement while N1 suggests regional lymph node metastasis.

Metastasis (M): Identifies the presence or absence of distant metastases. M0 indicates no distant metastasis, while M1 suggests cancer has spread to distant organs.

8.1.2 Grading with the Gleason Score:

The Gleason score is a fundamental component of categorization, assessing the aggressiveness of prostate cancer based on tissue examination. It combines two primary patterns seen in the biopsy specimen, with a higher score indicating a more aggressive tumor.

Grade Group 1-5: Introduced to simplify Gleason Scores into five categories. Grade Group 1 corresponds to Gleason Scores 6 or lower, while Grade Group 5 represents Gleason Scores 9-10.

Gleason scores are a grading system for prostate cancer. Medical pathologists set Gleason scores after studying tissue samples under a microscope.

Gleason scores range from 6 (low-grade cancer) to 10 (high-grade cancer). Low grade prostate cancer grows more slowly than high-grade cancer and is less likely to spread (metastasize). **Gleason score** is one of the ways healthcare providers classify prostate cancer as they develop treatment plans or set prognoses (what you can expect after treatment).

8.1.3 Grading with Gleason scores

Medical pathologists calculate Gleason scores by studying tissue samples under a microscope. If you have prostate cancer, your prostate tissues have cells that are mutating or changing from normal cells to abnormal or cancerous cells.

Early on, cancerous cells can masquerade as healthy cells. Over time, cancerous cells look less like healthy cells. Pathologists grade each tissue sample on a 1 to 5 scale. The lower the grade, the more cancer cells look like normal cells:

- Grade 1: The cancerous cells look a lot like normal cells.

- Grades 2-4: Cancerous cells in the tissue look less like normal cells.
- Grade 5: Cancerous cells look very abnormal.

Each area of prostate cancer may have a different grade, so pathologists pick the two areas that make up most of the cancer. They add the two areas' grades to come up with a Gleason score.

For example, if the largest area with cancer is Grade 3 and the next largest area is Grade 5, the Gleason score is 8. Any area with a combined Gleason score of 6 or higher is considered cancerous.

Your Gleason score doesn't rank potential ranges like ranges set for elevated PSA (prostate-specific antigen) tests. Instead, providers break Gleason scores into three categories:

- Gleason 6: The cells look like healthy cells, which is called well differentiated.
- Gleason 7: The cells look somewhat like healthy cells, which is called moderately differentiated.

- Gleason 8, 9 or 10: The cells look very different from healthy cells, which is called poorly differentiated or undifferentiated.

A Gleason score isn't good or bad, per se. Knowing your Gleason score is one way that healthcare providers predict how quickly prostate cancer might grow. Gleason scores range from 6 (low-grade cancer) to 10 (high-grade cancer). Low-grade prostate cancer grows more slowly than high-grade cancer and is less likely to spread (metastasize).

It's important to remember your Gleason score is just one of several pieces of information providers use to plan treatment or set a prognosis. They also consider the results of other tests and more biopsy information.

For example, when you had your biopsy, your healthcare provider obtained several samples or cores from your prostate. They checked how many cores had cancerous cells and whether most of the cells in the cores were cancerous cells. Other factors may include:

- Blood PSA level.
- Digital rectal exam results.
- Imaging test results like ultrasound, magnetic resonance imaging (MRI) or positron emission tomography (PET) scan.
- If there's cancer in both sides of your prostate.
- If prostate cancer spread to other areas of your body.

Gleason scores are a grading system for prostate cancer. Healthcare providers use Gleason score results to set up treatment plans. Gleason scores range from 6 (low-grade cancer) to 10 (high-grade cancer). But numbers don't tell the whole story about your prostate cancer. That story starts with your treatment plan and understanding what to expect from your treatment. Think of your Gleason score and other analysis as the next chapter in your story.

Talk to your healthcare provider any time you have questions about your Gleason score or any other test result. They'll be glad to help you understand what the numbers mean.

8.1.4 Impact on Treatment Decisions:

- Staging and grading inform treatment decisions, helping determine the appropriate interventions based on the cancer's characteristics.

- Treatment may range from active surveillance for low-risk cases to more aggressive approaches for advanced stages.

8.2 Risk Stratification of Prostate Cancer

Risk stratification is a crucial aspect of managing prostate cancer, guiding clinicians in tailoring treatment strategies based on the likelihood of disease progression and aggressiveness. This comprehensive exploration will delve into the low, intermediate, and high-risk categories, encompassing the parameters used for classification, prognostic factors, and the implications for treatment decisions.

Low, Intermediate, and High Risk Stratification:

Risk stratification categorizes prostate cancer into low, intermediate, and high-risk groups. This assessment considers factors such as PSA levels, Gleason score, and clinical stage. It guides treatment decisions, distinguishing between cases that may benefit from active surveillance, localized interventions, or more aggressive therapies.

8.2.1. Low-Risk Prostate Cancer:

a. Clinical Characteristics: Low-risk prostate cancer is characterized by features indicating a lower likelihood of aggressive behavior and progression.

- Gleason Score: Typically Gleason Score 6 or below, indicating well-differentiated cancer cells.

- PSA Level: Low PSA levels, often below 10 ng/mL.

- Clinical Stage: Limited to the prostate (T1 or T2).

b. Prognostic Implications: Favorable prognosis with a low risk of disease progression.

- Potential for active surveillance as a management strategy, avoiding immediate aggressive treatments.

c. Treatment Considerations: Active Surveillance: Regular monitoring with PSA tests, digital rectal exams, and periodic biopsies.

- Definitive Treatment: If progression is observed during surveillance, interventions such as surgery or radiation therapy may be considered.

8.2.2. Intermediate-Risk Prostate Cancer:

a. Clinical Characteristics: Intermediate-risk prostate cancer displays features between low and high-risk categories.

- Gleason Score: Often Gleason Score 7, indicating moderately differentiated cancer cells.

- PSA Level: Intermediate PSA levels, typically between 10 and 20 ng/mL.

- Clinical Stage: Extending beyond the prostate capsule but without distant metastasis (T2 or T3).

b. Prognostic Implications:

- Intermediate prognosis with a moderate risk of disease progression.

- Treatment decisions are influenced by factors such as age, overall health, and patient preferences.

c. Treatment Considerations:

- Options include radical prostatectomy, external beam radiation therapy, or brachytherapy.

- Androgen Deprivation Therapy (ADT) may be considered in certain cases.

8.2.3. High-Risk Prostate Cancer:

a. Clinical Characteristics:

- High-risk prostate cancer is associated with features indicating a higher likelihood of aggressive behavior.

- Gleason Score: Often Gleason Score 8 or above, indicating poorly differentiated cancer cells.

- PSA Level: Elevated PSA levels, frequently exceeding 20 ng/mL.

- Clinical Stage: Extensive local involvement or signs of regional lymph node involvement (T3 or T4).

b. Prognostic Implications:

- Unfavorable prognosis with a higher risk of disease progression and metastasis.

- Early and aggressive management is often warranted.

c. Treatment Considerations:

- Aggressive Treatment: Options may include radical prostatectomy, external beam radiation therapy, and androgen deprivation therapy (ADT).

- Combination Therapies: Some cases may benefit from a multimodal approach, combining surgery, radiation, and systemic therapies.

4. Evolving Concepts:

a. Genomic Profiling:

- Advances in genomic profiling provide additional insights into the molecular characteristics of prostate cancer.
- Genomic testing may refine risk stratification, aiding in personalized treatment decisions.

b. Shared Decision-Making:

- The approach to prostate cancer management increasingly involves shared decision-making between clinicians and patients.
- Patient preferences, overall health, and potential treatment side effects contribute to individualized care plans.

In conclusion, risk stratification is integral to the management of prostate cancer, guiding clinicians in selecting appropriate treatments based on the individual characteristics of the disease. The evolving landscape of prostate cancer care, incorporating genomic insights and shared decision-making, underscores the importance of tailoring interventions to optimize outcomes for patients across the spectrum of risk categories.

8.3. Clinical and Pathological Staging:

Combining clinical and pathological staging provides a comprehensive view. Clinical staging utilizes pre-treatment information, while pathological staging involves post-surgical evaluation. The integration of both aids in refining the categorization and treatment planning.

Clinical and Pathological Staging of Prostate Cancer: A Comprehensive Examination

Staging is a crucial aspect of understanding the extent and severity of prostate cancer, guiding treatment decisions and prognostic assessments.

This comprehensive exploration will delve into both clinical and pathological staging, outlining the key components, diagnostic tools, and implications for managing individuals with prostate cancer.

8.3.1. Clinical Staging:

a. Components:

Digital Rectal Examination (DRE): A physical examination where the healthcare provider assesses the size, shape, and consistency of the prostate through the rectum.

Prostate-Specific Antigen (PSA) Level: Blood tests measure PSA levels, providing an indication of prostate health.

Imaging Studies: Techniques such as transrectal ultrasound, magnetic resonance imaging (MRI), and computed tomography (CT) scans help visualize the prostate and surrounding tissues.

b. TNM System:

- The TNM system classifies tumors based on T (tumor size and extent), N (lymph node involvement), and M (metastasis) categories.
- T categories range from T1 (small, confined tumors) to T4 (tumors extending into adjacent structures).

c. Clinical Stage Groups:

Stage I: T1 or T2, low PSA levels, no evidence of spread beyond the prostate.

Stage II: T1 or T2, higher PSA levels, or T3, tumor extends beyond the prostate.

Stage III: T4 or involvement of nearby tissues.

Stage IV: Spread to lymph nodes (N1) or distant metastasis (M1).

d. Limitations:

- Clinical staging may have limitations in accurately assessing the full extent of the disease, particularly regarding lymph node involvement and microscopic spread.

8.3.2. Pathological Staging:

a. Components:

Gleason Score: Microscopic examination of prostate tissue assigns a Gleason Score based on the appearance of cancer cells, ranging from 6 (well-differentiated) to 10 (poorly differentiated).

Surgical Pathology: Tissue obtained through biopsy or surgery provides information on the size, location, and characteristics of the tumor.

Lymph Node Involvement: Examining lymph nodes removed during surgery determines if cancer has spread.

b. TNM System: The pathological TNM system refines the clinical staging based on the actual findings from surgery or biopsy. Pathological staging includes additional details on tumor characteristics.

c. Pathological Stage Groups:

Stage I: T1 or T2, Gleason Score 6 or lower, confined to the prostate.

Stage II: T1 or T2, Gleason Score 7, tumor may extend beyond the prostate.

Stage III: T3 or T4, or N1 (lymph node involvement).

Stage IV: M1 (distant metastasis).

d. Prognostic Significance: Pathological staging provides more accurate information for predicting the risk of recurrence and guiding treatment decisions.

8.3.3. Integrating Clinical and Pathological Staging:

a. Multidisciplinary Assessment: Treatment decisions often involve a multidisciplinary team, considering both clinical and pathological staging. The collaborative approach helps tailor interventions based on the specific characteristics of the disease.

b. Post-Treatment Evaluation: Post-treatment, monitoring PSA levels and potential recurrence is essential to assess treatment efficacy and guide further management.

c. Advances in Imaging: Advanced imaging technologies, such as multiparametric MRI, contribute to improved preoperative staging, aiding in surgical planning.

The combination of clinical and pathological staging provides a comprehensive understanding of prostate cancer, assisting healthcare professionals in determining optimal treatment strategies and offering prognostic insights. Advances in diagnostic tools and collaborative approaches continue to refine the staging process, contributing to more personalized and effective management of individuals with prostate cancer.

8.4. Localized and Advanced Stages of Prostate Cancer

Prostate cancer classification into localized or advanced stages is pivotal for treatment planning, prognosis, and guiding therapeutic decisions. This extensive exploration will delve into the criteria, diagnostic methods, and implications associated with categorizing prostate cancer into localized and advanced stages.

Localized vs. Advanced Prostate Cancer:
Categorizing prostate cancer as localized or advanced depends on its extent beyond the prostate. Localized cases are confined to the prostate, while advanced cases may involve nearby tissues, lymph nodes, or distant organs.

8.4.1. Localized Prostate Cancer:
a. Criteria: Localized prostate cancer is confined to the prostate gland without evidence of spread beyond its boundaries. Typically identified during

early stages through screening methods like PSA tests, digital rectal exams (DRE), and prostate biopsies.

b. Diagnostic Methods:
PSA Levels: Low to moderately elevated PSA levels may indicate the presence of localized disease.
Gleason Score: Gleason Score 6 or below suggests well-differentiated, less aggressive cancer cells.
Clinical Staging (TNM): T1 or T2 stages, indicating tumors that are still within the prostate.

c. Treatment Options:
Active Surveillance: For low-risk cases, monitoring through regular PSA tests, DRE, and periodic biopsies may be employed.

Definitive Treatments: Options include surgery (radical prostatectomy) and radiation therapy, aiming to eradicate the localized tumor.

d. Prognosis:
- Localized prostate cancer often carries a favorable prognosis, especially when detected early and managed appropriately.

8.4.2. Advanced Prostate Cancer:
a. Criteria: prostate cancer indicates the presence of more aggressive disease with potential spread beyond the prostate.
- May involve invasion into surrounding tissues, lymph node involvement, or distant metastasis.

b. Diagnostic Methods:
PSA Levels: Higher PSA levels, especially in the context of a rising trend, may raise suspicion of advanced disease.
Gleason Score: Scores above 7, indicating more poorly differentiated and aggressive cancer cells.

Clinical Staging (TNM): T3 or T4 stages, lymph node involvement (N1), or distant metastasis (M1).

c. Treatment Options:

Systemic Therapies: Androgen deprivation therapy (ADT) or hormone therapy to suppress testosterone and slow cancer growth.

Chemotherapy: Utilized in certain cases, especially if the cancer has become resistant to hormonal treatments.

Targeted Therapies: Emerging approaches targeting specific pathways involved in cancer progression.

d. Prognosis: Advanced prostate cancer carries a more guarded prognosis due to the potential for metastasis and challenges in complete eradication.

8.4.3. Transition States:

a. Biochemical Recurrence: Some cases may experience a rise in PSA levels after initial treatment, indicating biochemical recurrence. This does not necessarily equate to clinical progression, and decisions about further interventions depend on various factors.

b. Castration-Resistant Prostate Cancer (CRPC): This occurs when prostate cancer progresses despite low testosterone levels achieved through ADT. It also signifies a transition to a more aggressive state, often requiring different treatment modalities.

8.4.4. Challenges and Advances:

a. Imaging Technologies: Advanced imaging, such as multiparametric MRI and positron emission tomography (PET) scans, aids in detecting the extent of disease and guiding treatment decisions.

b. Personalized Approaches: The era of precision medicine involves tailoring treatments based on the molecular characteristics of the cancer, enhancing the ability to address advanced disease.

Therefore, categorizing prostate cancer into localized or advanced stages is pivotal for informing treatment decisions and predicting outcomes. Advances in diagnostic methods and treatment modalities contribute to a more nuanced understanding of the disease, allowing for personalized and effective management strategies tailored to the specific characteristics of each case.

PART B

Prostate cancer treatment

Prostate cancer treatment

You probably never think about your prostate. Until a routine screening test says you might have something to worry about. And if it turns out you might have prostate cancer, life could feel like it's spinning out of control. It's OK (and natural) to have all sorts of emotions when you're trying to process this kind of news.

Early-stage prostate cancer rarely causes symptoms. As the cancer progresses, you might need to pee more often, or find it harder to completely empty your bladder. It might be painful to pee or to ejaculate, and you might have blood in your semen or pee. You might have pain in your lower back, hip and chest and numbness in your feet and legs. If you have any of these symptoms, it's important to see a healthcare provider right away. Your provider will start off by asking about your symptoms and your medical history. If they suspect you have cancer, they might do a few different tests, like a <u>prostate exam</u>, to confirm your diagnosis and find out how big and how quickly your cancer is growing (what stage it is). Your provider might also do one or more of these tests:

Digital rectal exam

Your provider will check out your prostate bumps or hard areas on your prostate gland. They'll do this by inserting a gloved, lubricated finger (digit) into your rectum to reach your prostate.

Prostate-specific antigen (PSA) blood test:

This test shows if your prostate is making higher-than-normal levels of PSA. <u>Elevated PSA levels</u> could mean you have cancer.

Biopsy

Your provider will use a needle to take a small amount of tissue from your prostate and send it to our lab where a pathologist will look at it under a microscope. A <u>biopsy</u> will tell for sure if you have prostate cancer.

Meet Your Healthcare providers from different specialties will work closely together to plan your personalized treatment based on your values, priorities, tolerance for side effects and desired quality of life. Your care team could include:

- Urologists.
- Oncologists.
- Radiologists (imaging specialists).
- Pathologists (body tissue specialists).
- Anesthesiologists.
- Social workers.
- Nurse practitioners.
- Physician assistants.

If you are confirm to have prostate cancer, the health worker will decide what type of treatment (if any) will be the most effective for you. Because prostate cancer grows slowly, you might never need treatment. But if you do, there's good news — most prostate cancers are highly curable. Here are a few of the treatment options your health provider might recommend:

CHAPTER 9

Active Surveillance for Prostate Cancer

Active Surveillance (AS) has emerged as a thoughtful and increasingly utilized approach in managing prostate cancer, particularly for cases with low-risk characteristics. This extensive exploration delves into the intricacies of Active Surveillance as a treatment option, covering its principles, patient selection criteria, monitoring protocols, psychological aspects, and the evolving landscape of this conservative management strategy.

9.1 Principles of Active Surveillance:

Active Surveillance is a strategy designed to closely monitor low-risk prostate cancer without immediate intervention. The primary goal is to avoid overtreatment in cases where the cancer is slow-growing and poses a low risk of progression.

9.1.1 Rationale for Active Surveillance: Active Surveillance is employed for low-risk prostate cancer cases, where the cancer is deemed to be slow-growing and unlikely to cause harm during a patient's natural lifespan. The primary goal is to avoid unnecessary interventions, such as surgery or radiation, that may pose risks of side effects.

Monitoring Protocols: Active Surveillance involves regular monitoring through a combination of PSA tests, digital rectal examinations (DRE), and periodic biopsies. Imaging studies, such as multiparametric MRI, may also be employed to assess any changes in the prostate over time.

9.2 Patient Selection Criteria

Candidates for Active Surveillance typically have low-risk prostate cancer, characterized by a Gleason score of 6 or lower, low PSA levels, and limited tumor volume clinical stage T1 or T2 tumors. The decision to pursue AS is individualized, considering the patient's age, overall health, and personal preferences.

Shared Decision-Making: The decision to embark on Active Surveillance is a shared process between the patient and the healthcare team. Detailed discussions about the potential risks and benefits, as well as the psychological impact, help in making informed decisions aligned with the patient's values and preferences.

Patient Adherence and Satisfaction: Patient adherence to Active Surveillance protocols is crucial. Urologists work closely with patients to ensure regular follow-ups and address any concerns. Patient satisfaction with this approach is often high, especially among those who avoid unnecessary side effects associated with more aggressive treatments.

9.3 Criteria for Transition to Treatment:

Specific triggers may prompt a transition from Active Surveillance to active treatment. These can include changes in PSA velocity, an increase in Gleason score on biopsy, or other indications suggesting a shift from low to higher-risk disease.

Risk Reclassification and Transition to Treatment: If there are indications that the cancer is progressing, such as a rise in PSA levels or changes in biopsy results, the patient may be reclassified as higher risk. At this point, a transition to more active treatment options, such as surgery or radiation therapy, may be recommended.

Evolving Landscape: Active Surveillance protocols continue to evolve with advancements in imaging and biomarker technologies. Multiparametric MRI is increasingly used to enhance the accuracy of monitoring, providing more detailed insights into the prostate and potentially reducing the need for repeat biopsies.

Advancements in Monitoring Technologies: Ongoing advancements in monitoring technologies, such as improved imaging modalities and biomarker assessments, contribute to refining the Active Surveillance approach. These innovations enhance the precision of risk assessment and further tailor monitoring strategies.

Integration into Multidisciplinary Care: Active Surveillance is an integral part of multidisciplinary prostate cancer care. Collaboration between urologists, oncologists, radiologists, and support staff ensures a holistic approach, considering both the medical and psychosocial aspects of patient care

9.4 Psychological Aspects:

Active Surveillance brings unique psychological considerations. Patients may experience anxiety about the uncertainty of cancer progression. Robust support systems, counseling, and clear communication from healthcare professionals play a vital role in addressing these concerns.

Psychosocial Support and Education: Patients opting for Active Surveillance benefit from comprehensive psychosocial support and education. Urologists and healthcare teams ensure that patients understand the nature of their cancer, the rationale behind Active Surveillance, and the potential risks and benefits. This approach fosters shared decision-making and helps alleviate anxiety.

Long-Term Outcomes:

Studies evaluating the long-term outcomes of Active Surveillance demonstrate that for appropriately selected patients, the approach is associated with favorable outcomes. Many patients on Active Surveillance may never require definitive treatment, while those who do transition to treatment often do so with curative intent.

Quality of Life Considerations:

Active Surveillance is often associated with a favorable impact on quality of life, as it avoids the potential side effects of immediate treatment. Patients on AS may experience fewer complications related to surgery or radiation, contributing to a better overall quality of life. Active Surveillance prioritizes maintaining the patient's quality of life. By avoiding immediate invasive treatments, individuals on Active Surveillance can maintain normal urinary and sexual function. This approach acknowledges that not all prostate cancers warrant aggressive interventions.

9.5 Research and Future Directions:

Ongoing research explores refinements in patient selection, monitoring strategies, and the incorporation of novel biomarkers. The aim is to further optimize Active Surveillance protocols and expand its application to a broader range of patients.

Active Surveillance has emerged as a valuable and patient-centric option for managing low-risk prostate cancer. Balancing the benefits of avoiding immediate treatment-related side effects with the need for vigilant monitoring, Active Surveillance reflects a personalized and evolving approach in the dynamic landscape of prostate cancer care. Continuous research and patient-centered initiatives contribute to the ongoing enhancement of Active Surveillance protocols, shaping the future of prostate cancer management.

9.6 Facts about active surveillance

Active Surveillance is not a treatment aimed at curing prostate cancer but rather a strategy for monitoring low-risk cases without immediate intervention. The goal of Active Surveillance is to avoid unnecessary treatments, such as surgery or radiation therapy, which can have associated side effects. Instead, it involves regular monitoring through PSA tests, digital rectal exams, and periodic prostate biopsies to track the progression of the disease.

If, during the course of Active Surveillance, there are indications that the cancer is progressing, the healthcare team may reconsider the treatment approach. At that point, a shift to more active treatments, such as surgery or radiation therapy, might be recommended to address the advancing cancer. Active surveillanceit seeks to balance the potential risks and benefits of treatment, ensuring that patients receive interventions only when necessary.

The decision to transition to a curative treatment depends on the specific characteristics of the cancer, changes in monitoring results, and the collaborative decision-making between the patient and their healthcare team.

The goal of Active Surveillance is to avoid unnecessary treatment in cases where the cancer is low-risk and unlikely to progress significantly. It is not intended as a curative approach but rather a strategy to balance disease control with minimizing treatment-related side effects.

If there is evidence of disease progression or a change in risk factors during Active Surveillance, the healthcare team may consider transitioning to curative treatment options. Common curative treatments for prostate cancer include: Prostatectomy, Radiation Therapy, Cryotherapy, Hormone Therapy, Focal Therapy:

9.7 Curative Treatments for Prostate Cancer

1. **Prostatectomy (Surgery):** Surgical removal of the prostate gland. The purpose of the procedure is to eliminates the primary tumor and is considered curative if the cancer is confined to the prostate.

2. Radiation Therapy: High-energy beams are used to target and kill cancer cells. This radiation Destroys cancer cells and may be employed as external beam radiation or brachytherapy (internal radiation).

3. Cryotherapy: Freezing of prostate tissue to destroy cancer cells. Cryotherapy targets and eliminates cancer cells within the prostate.

4. Hormone Therapy: Medications to suppress or block the effects of male hormones. Purpose of hormone therapy is to slow down the growth of prostate cancer cells, often used in combination with other treatments.

5. Focal Therapy: Targeted treatment of specific areas within the prostate. Focal therapy aims to treat localized tumors while preserving healthy prostate tissue.

Each patient's situation is unique, and treatment decisions are tailored to individual circumstances.

Regular follow-ups, including PSA tests, digital rectal examinations, and possibly repeat biopsies, are essential components of Active Surveillance to ensure timely detection of any progression. If progression occurs, the healthcare team will discuss appropriate curative treatment options with the patient. Active Surveillance for prostate cancer typically involves monitoring the disease rather than administering specific medications for treatment.

9.8 Medications for Managing Prostate Cancer

Medications may be prescribed to manage certain aspects of prostate cancer or its potential side effects. Here are some medications that might be considered in the context of Active Surveillance:

1. 5-alpha reductase inhibitors (e.g., finasteride, dutasteride): These medications can reduce the size of the prostate and lower PSA levels. While not directly treating prostate cancer, they may impact disease progression and help manage urinary symptoms.

2. Anti-androgens (e.g., bicalutamide, flutamide): Anti-androgens can block the effects of male hormones (androgens) on prostate cells. They are sometimes used in combination with other treatments or as part of intermittent androgen deprivation therapy.

3. Bone-strengthening medications (e.g., bisphosphonates, denosumab): Prostate cancer can sometimes spread to the bones. These medications are used to strengthen bones and reduce the risk of complications related to bone metastases.

4. GnRH agonists (e.g., leuprolide, goserelin): These medications reduce the production of testosterone, slowing down the growth of prostate cancer cells. They are commonly used in more advanced stages but may be considered in certain cases during Active Surveillance.

It's essential to note that the choice of medications and the decision to use them during Active Surveillance will depend on the specific characteristics of the prostate cancer, the patient's overall health, and the recommendations of the healthcare team.

CHAPTER 10

Treatment for Prostate Cancer

10.1 Prostatectomy

Prostatectomy is a surgical procedure involving the removal of the prostate gland, commonly employed as a treatment for prostate cancer. This extensive exploration delves into the nuances of prostatectomy, encompassing the different types, surgical techniques, considerations, and postoperative care.

Introduction to Prostatectomy:

Prostatectomy is a curative surgical intervention designed to eliminate cancerous tissue within the prostate. The procedure is indicated for localized prostate cancer and may be considered in cases where the cancer is confined to the prostate gland.

10.1.1 Types of Prostatectomy:

There are several types of prostatectomy, each with its unique approach:

Radical Prostatectomy: Removal of the entire prostate gland, seminal vesicles, and surrounding tissues.

Simple Prostatectomy: Partial removal of the prostate, typically used for benign prostatic hyperplasia (BPH) rather than cancer.

Radical Prostatectomy

During radical prostatectomy, the surgeon removes the entire prostate gland, seminal vesicles, and nearby tissues. Lymph nodes may also be sampled for evaluation. The goal is to achieve complete removal while preserving the surrounding structure

Types of Radical Prostatectomy:

Open Radical Prostatectomy: Involves a traditional surgical approach with a single, larger incision.

Laparoscopic Radical Prostatectomy: Utilizes minimally invasive techniques with smaller incisions and the assistance of a camera for visualization.

Robotic-Assisted Radical Prostatectomy: Incorporates robotic technology to enhance precision, flexibility, and visualization during the procedure.

Indications for Radical Prostatectomy: Radical prostatectomy is typically recommended when prostate cancer is localized and has not metastasized. Factors such as the Gleason score,

PSA levels, and clinical stage influence the decision for this surgical intervention.

Preoperative Considerations:
Before the surgery, patients undergo a comprehensive evaluation, including imaging studies, blood tests, and discussions about potential risks and benefits. Counseling sessions address expectations, potential side effects, and the impact on urinary continence and sexual function.

Radical Prostatectomy Procedure:
Anesthetic Administration: The patient is placed under general anesthesia.
Incision: Depending on the chosen approach (open, laparoscopic, or robotic-assisted), incisions are made to access the prostate.
Removal of Prostate: The entire prostate gland, along with nearby tissues, is carefully removed. Lymph nodes may also be sampled for evaluation.
Preservation of Nerves: Efforts may be made to preserve nerves responsible for erectile function to

minimize the risk of postoperative sexual dysfunction.

Closure: The surgical site is meticulously closed, and drainage tubes may be inserted to manage fluids.

Radical prostatectomy is a significant and effective intervention for localized prostate cancer. Whether performed through an open, laparoscopic, or robotic-assisted approach, the surgery requires careful consideration of individual patient factors. Continuous advancements in surgical technology contribute to optimizing outcomes and preserving the quality of life for individuals undergoing radical prostatectomy.

Simple Prostatectomy:

Simple prostatectomy is a surgical procedure primarily used to treat benign prostatic hyperplasia (BPH), a non-cancerous enlargement of the prostate gland. Unlike radical prostatectomy, which is employed for prostate cancer, simple prostatectomy involves the removal of only a portion of the prostate gland. This extensive exploration delves into the various aspects of simple prostatectomy, encompassing indications, surgical techniques, considerations, and postoperative care.

Introduction to Simple Prostatectomy: Simple prostatectomy is a surgical intervention designed to alleviate symptoms associated with an enlarged prostate, such as urinary difficulties. It is a common treatment for benign prostatic hyperplasia (BPH), a condition prevalent in aging men.

Indications for Simple Prostatectomy:
Simple prostatectomy is indicated when BPH causes significant urinary obstruction, recurrent urinary tract infections, or fails to respond adequately to conservative treatments. It is not typically employed for prostate cancer.

Preoperative Considerations:

Before the surgery, patients undergo a thorough evaluation, including urodynamic studies, imaging studies, and discussions about potential risks and benefits. Preoperative counseling addresses expectations and potential side effects.

Surgical Techniques:

Simple prostatectomy can be performed through different techniques, including:

Open Simple Prostatectomy: A traditional surgical approach with an incision made in the lower abdomen to access and remove the enlarged part of the prostate.

Laparoscopic Simple Prostatectomy: Utilizes minimally invasive techniques with smaller incisions and a camera for visualization.

Robotic-Assisted Simple Prostatectomy: Incorporates robotic technology for enhanced precision and maneuverability.

Simple Prostatectomy Procedure:

During the procedure, the surgeon removes the enlarged portion of the prostate, leaving the rest of the gland intact. This allows for relief of urinary obstruction while preserving prostate function.

10.1.2 Postoperative Care:

After prostatectomy, patients typically stay in the hospital for a brief period. Recovery involves managing pain, monitoring for potential complications, and gradually resuming normal activities. Patients are advised on pelvic floor exercises to support continence and erectile function.

10.1.3 Urinary Continence and Sexual Function:

Prostatectomy can impact urinary continence and sexual function. Recovery varies among individuals, and patients are supported through postoperative care, including rehabilitation and discussions about potential interventions for erectile dysfunction.

10.1.4 Follow-Up and Monitoring:
Regular follow-up appointments include PSA tests, digital rectal examinations, and possibly imaging studies to monitor for any signs of recurrence. Ongoing care addresses potential long-term effects and ensures comprehensive postoperative management.

10.1.5 Advancements in Prostatectomy:
Advances in surgical techniques, including robotic-assisted surgery, have contributed to reduced invasiveness, shorter recovery times, and improved outcomes. Research continues to refine surgical approaches and enhance patient outcomes.

Prostatectomy stands as a cornerstone in the comprehensive treatment of localized prostate cancer. Whether performed through open, laparoscopic, or robotic-assisted techniques, the procedure requires careful consideration of individual patient factors. Advances in surgical technology and postoperative care contribute to optimizing outcomes and preserving the quality of life for individuals undergoing prostatectomy. Continuous research and multidisciplinary collaboration further shape the landscape of prostate cancer treatment, ensuring that prostatectomy remains a vital component in the pursuit of effective, patient-centered care.

Simple prostatectomy is a valuable intervention for managing the symptoms of benign prostatic hyperplasia, providing relief from urinary obstruction. Whether performed through open, laparoscopic, or robotic-assisted techniques, the surgery requires careful consideration of individual patient factors. Continuous advancements in surgical technology contribute to optimizing outcomes and preserving the quality of life for individuals undergoing simple prostatectomy.

10.2 RADIATION THERAPY

Radiation Therapy in the Treatment of Prostate Cancer: Prostate cancer is a prevalent malignancy affecting men worldwide, and radiation therapy stands as a pivotal modality in its comprehensive management. This extensive exploration delves into the multifaceted aspects of radiation therapy, covering its types, treatment planning, side effects, and technological advances.

10.2.1 Types of Radiation Therapy: Three types of radiation therapy in treatment of prostate cancer includes:
- External Beam Radiation,
- Brachytherapy and
- Proton Beam Therapy

External Beam Radiation:

External Beam Radiation in the Treatment of Prostate Cancer: Prostate cancer, a prevalent malignancy affecting men, often necessitates a multidimensional approach for effective management. External Beam Radiation (EBRT) stands out as a fundamental modality, offering targeted radiation to prostate tumors while sparing surrounding healthy tissues. This approach delivers precisely targeted radiation from outside the body to the prostate. Here, Patients undergo daily sessions over several weeks, ensuring gradual and accurate radiation exposure

The three techniques of external beam radiation includes:

i) Conventional (2D) Radiation Therapy:

ii) Three-Dimensional Conformal Radiation Therapy (3D-CRT):

iii) Intensity-Modulated Radiation Therapy (IMRT):

i) Conventional (2D) Radiation Therapy: Traditional technique utilizing two-dimensional imaging for treatment planning. In this procedure, radiation beams are directed at the prostate from various angles. Using this techniques minimize exposure to healthy tissues.

ii) Three-Dimensional Conformal Radiation Therapy (3D-CRT): Advances from 2D, incorporating 3D imaging to shape radiation beams. **Procedure for 3D-CRT** enables precise targeting of the prostate, minimizing irradiation of adjacent structures. **Benefits of 3D-CRT includes**: improved accuracy, reducing side effects compared to conventional techniques.

iii) Intensity-Modulated Radiation Therapy (IMRT):
Employs computer-controlled modulators to vary radiation intensity across multiple beam angles. **This Procedure** Optimized dose distribution, shaping beams to the contours of the prostate. **The Benefits** of this procedure is to enhance precision in delivering higher doses to the tumor while sparing healthy tissues. Generally External Beam Radiation is Effective in treating localized tumors, although potential side effects such as fatigue and urinary changes may arise.

Brachytherapy:

Brachytherapy in the Treatment of Prostate Cancer:

Involves implanting radioactive seeds directly into the prostate tissue.

Seeds emit radiation over time, providing localized treatment with minimal impact on surrounding tissues.

Benefits and Considerations: High dose to the tumor, shorter treatment duration, but potential for urinary and sexual side effects.

A Comprehensive Exploration

Prostate cancer management has evolved, and Brachytherapy, an intricate form of radiation therapy, has emerged as a vital modality in the therapeutic arsenal. This extensive examination delves into the nuanced aspects of Brachytherapy, encompassing its techniques, patient selection, side effects, and the evolving landscape of technological advancements.

1. Techniques of Brachytherapy:

i) Low-Dose Rate (LDR) Brachytherapy: This Involves the permanent implantation of radioactive seeds directly into the prostate.

Procedure: Seeds emit a continuous, low dose of radiation over an extended period. LDR Provides a localized and sustained dose to the tumor, minimizing impact on surrounding healthy **tissues.**

ii). High-Dose Rate (HDR) Brachytherapy: Delivers a high dose of radiation temporarily through catheters inserted into the prostate.

Procedure: Catheters are precisely positioned, and a remote-controlled machine administers the radiation. HDR enables targeted, intensified radiation while minimizing radiation exposure to adjacent structures.

c. Permanent vs. Temporary Brachytherapy: LDR Brachytherapy involves permanent seed implantation, while HDR Brachytherapy is temporary.

Procedure: Permanent seeds remain in the prostate, whereas temporary catheters are removed after the treatment session. The choice of either permanent or temporary Brachytherapy depends on patient and tumor characteristics, with both techniques demonstrating efficacy.

2. Patient Selection and Planning:

a. Eligibility Criteria: Suitable for patients with localized prostate cancer, typically with a low or intermediate risk profile.

Selection Factors: Consideration of tumor stage, patient health, and preferences.

Benefits and Considerations: Offers a curative option for eligible patients with favorable risk features.

b. Treatment Planning: Precise planning ensures optimal distribution of radiation to the prostate while sparing nearby structures.

Imaging Techniques: CT and ultrasound assist in visualizing the prostate and guiding seed or catheter placement.

Benefits and Considerations: Tailored plans aim to maximize tumor coverage and minimize radiation to healthy tissues.

c. Combined Modalities: Brachytherapy may be combined with External Beam Radiation for enhanced therapeutic effect.

Procedure: External beam radiation provides supplemental treatment to areas beyond the reach of brachytherapy.

Benefits and Considerations: Comprehensive approach targeting both localized and potentially microscopic disease.

3. Side Effects and Management:

a. **Short-Term Side Effects:** Common effects include temporary urinary changes, mild discomfort, and potential fatigue.

Management: Supportive care measures, including medications to alleviate symptoms.

Impact on Quality of Life: Generally transient, with most side effects resolving post-treatment.

b. Long-Term Side Effects: Potential long-term effects may include urinary changes and, rarely, sexual dysfunction.

Management: Ongoing monitoring and interventions, including medications or lifestyle modifications.

Impact on Quality of Life: Varied, with advancements aiming to minimize long-term effects.

c. **Post-Brachytherapy Imaging**: Follow-up imaging, such as MRI or CT scans, assesses treatment response and potential recurrence.

Procedure: Imaging helps evaluate the prostate's condition and identify any areas of concern.

Benefits and Considerations: Monitoring aids in timely interventions if needed and provides reassurance to patients.

4. Advances in Brachytherapy:
    a. **Real-Time Planning and Imaging**:

Incorporates real-time planning and imaging during the procedure for enhanced precision. Technological Aspects of Brachytherapy includes advanced imaging modalities that improve seed or catheter placement accuracy.

Clinical Benefits: Improved visualization ensures optimal radiation distribution, reducing the risk of complications.

b. Focal Brachytherapy

Targets specific regions of the prostate, sparing healthy tissue.

Procedure: Involves precise seed placement or catheter positioning based on tumor characteristics.

Benefits and Considerations: Minimizes impact on surrounding structures, potentially reducing side effects.

c. Salvage Brachytherapy:

Utilized in cases of recurrent prostate cancer after initial treatment.

Procedure: Involves implanting additional seeds or delivering a higher dose through catheters.

Benefits and Considerations: Salvage brachytherapy offers a curative option for select patients with recurrent disease.

In conclusion, Brachytherapy serves as a dynamic and effective treatment modality for prostate cancer. The diverse techniques, meticulous patient selection, management of side effects, and ongoing technological advancements collectively contribute to improved outcomes and enhanced quality of life for individuals undergoing brachytherapy for prostate cancer.

c. Proton Beam Therapy:

Utilizes proton beams for precise radiation delivery, minimizing damage to surrounding tissues. It Requires specialized facilities, and the treatment course is similar to external beam radiation.

Benefits and Considerations: Reduced radiation exposure to healthy tissues, though limited availability of proton therapy centers.

Proton Beam Therapy in the Treatment of Prostate Cancer: An In-Depth Analysis

Prostate cancer treatment has witnessed a paradigm shift with the advent of Proton Beam Therapy (PBT), a sophisticated form of radiation therapy. This comprehensive exploration delves into the nuanced aspects of PBT, encompassing its principles, advantages, patient selection, side effects, and the evolving landscape of technological advancements.

1. Principles of Proton Beam Therapy:
a. Particle Physics Basis:

Protons, charged particles, are utilized to deliver precise radiation to cancerous tissues.

Mechanism: Protons deposit their maximum energy at the tumor site, known as the Bragg peak, minimizing damage to surrounding healthy tissues.

Benefits and Considerations: Enhanced precision in targeting tumors, reducing radiation exposure to adjacent organs.

b. Treatment Planning:

Requires meticulous treatment planning to exploit the advantages of proton beams.

Imaging Techniques: CT scans and advanced imaging modalities aid in visualizing the prostate for precise treatment planning.

Benefits and Considerations: Tailored plans aim to maximize tumor coverage while sparing healthy tissues.

Advantages of Proton Beam Therapy:

a. Tissue-Sparing Effect: Protons deposit most of their energy at the tumor site, minimizing damage to healthy tissues.

Clinical Benefits: Reduces the risk of long-term side effects associated with radiation exposure to adjacent structures.

Considerations: Particularly advantageous for tumors located near critical structures.

b. Reduced Radiation to Surrounding Organs:

Proton beams allow for precise control of radiation delivery, sparing nearby organs.

Clinical Benefits: Lower doses to organs such as the bladder and rectum, potentially reducing side effects.

Considerations: May contribute to improved quality of life during and post-treatment.

c. Pediatric Applications:

PBT is particularly beneficial for pediatric patients due to its ability to spare normal tissues.

Clinical Benefits: Reduces the risk of secondary cancers and developmental issues in pediatric populations.

Considerations: Proton therapy is increasingly used in pediatric oncology for various tumor types.

3. Patient Selection and Planning:
a. Eligibility Criteria:

Suitable for a variety of prostate cancer cases, particularly those near critical structures.

Selection Factors: Tumor characteristics, patient health, and preferences are considered.

Benefits and Considerations: Offers a curative option with potential advantages for select patient profiles.

b. Treatment Planning:

Precise planning is crucial to exploit the advantages of proton beams.

Imaging Techniques: CT scans and advanced imaging modalities aid in visualizing the prostate for precise treatment planning.

Benefits and Considerations: Tailored plans aim to maximize tumor coverage while sparing healthy tissues.

4. Side Effects and Management:

a. Short-Term Side Effects:

Common effects include temporary fatigue, mild skin irritation, and potential gastrointestinal discomfort.

Management: Supportive care measures, including rest and symptom-specific medications.

Impact on Quality of Life: Generally transient, with most side effects resolving post-treatment.

b. Long-Term Side Effects:
Potential long-term effects may include urinary changes and, rarely, sexual dysfunction.

Management: Ongoing monitoring and interventions, including medications or lifestyle modifications.

Impact on Quality of Life: Varied, with advancements aiming to minimize long-term effects.

5. Advances in Proton Beam Therapy:

a. Pencil Beam Scanning: Utilizes narrow proton beams that can be precisely controlled, enhancing treatment precision.

Technological Aspects: Advanced scanning technology allows for detailed modulation of the proton beam.

Clinical Benefits: Improved conformity to tumor shape, reducing exposure to nearby healthy tissues.

b. Integrated Imaging:

Real-time imaging during treatment sessions enhances precision and accuracy.

Technological Aspects: Integration of imaging technologies into treatment machines.

Clinical Benefits: Improved targeting and verification, reducing the risk of errors during treatment.

c. Hypofractionation Protocols:

Investigates the use of fewer treatment sessions with higher doses per session.

Clinical Trials: Ongoing studies explore the efficacy and safety of hypofractionation in prostate cancer.

Considerations: May offer a more convenient treatment schedule for patients.

In conclusion Proton Beam Therapy represents a groundbreaking approach in the management of prostate cancer, capitalizing on its unique physical properties to enhance treatment precision and reduce side effects. The dynamic interplay between particle physics principles, clinical advantages, patient selection criteria, and ongoing technological innovations positions PBT as a forefront modality in the evolving landscape of prostate cancer treatment.

10.2.2. Treatment Planning and Simulation:

a. Imaging and Targeting: Advanced imaging techniques such as MRI and CT aid in precise prostate localization.

Procedure: Simulation sessions determine optimal radiation angles and patient positioning.

Benefits and Considerations: Enhanced targeting reduces damage to adjacent organs, improving treatment accuracy.

b. Dose Calculation and Optimization:

Dosimetrists calculate the radiation dose to ensure maximum tumor exposure.

Procedure: Treatment plans are tailored based on tumor characteristics and proximity to critical structures.

Benefits and Considerations: Optimization aims to maximize cancer cell destruction while minimizing damage to healthy tissue.

c. Treatment Verification:

Daily imaging or monitoring during treatment sessions ensures accurate radiation delivery.

Procedure: Varied verification methods, including image-guided radiation therapy (IGRT) or real-time tracking.

Benefits and Considerations: Reduces the risk of errors, enhancing treatment precision and efficacy.

Treatment Planning and Simulation in Radiation Therapy for Prostate Cancer: An In-Depth Exploration

Effective treatment planning and simulation are critical components of radiation therapy for prostate cancer, ensuring precise delivery of therapeutic doses while minimizing exposure to surrounding healthy tissues. This comprehensive examination delves into the nuanced aspects of treatment planning and simulation, covering techniques, imaging modalities, quality assurance, and the evolving landscape of technological advancements.

10.2.3 Importance of Treatment Planning:

a. Precision in Dose Delivery: Treatment planning aims to maximize radiation to the prostate while sparing nearby critical structures.

Technological Advances: Advanced planning software allows for intricate calculations and optimization.

Benefits and Considerations: Achieving a therapeutic dose to the tumor while minimizing toxicity to adjacent organs.

b. Individualized Patient Plans: Each patient's anatomy and tumor characteristics are unique, requiring personalized treatment plans.

Customization Factors: Consideration of tumor size, location, and proximity to organs at risk.

Benefits and Considerations: Tailored plans optimize treatment outcomes and reduce potential side effects.

10.2.4 Imaging Modalities in Treatment Planning:

a. **Computed Tomography (CT)**: CT scans provide detailed anatomical information for treatment planning.

Procedure: Patients undergo CT simulation in the treatment position to ensure accurate representation.

Benefits and Considerations: Precise visualization aids in delineating the prostate and surrounding structures.

b. **Magnetic Resonance Imaging (MRI)**: MRI complements CT scans, offering superior soft tissue contrast.

Integration in Planning: Fusion of MRI with CT data refines tumor delineation and enhances accuracy.

Benefits and Considerations: Improved visualization of the prostate and nearby organs for more precise planning.

c. Positron Emission Tomography (PET): PET scans may be utilized for functional imaging and to identify areas of increased metabolic activity.

Integration in Planning: Combining PET with CT provides comprehensive information for tumor delineation.

Benefits and Considerations: Helps in identifying areas of potential tumor spread or recurrence.

10.2.5. Simulation Sessions:

a. Patient Positioning: Accurate simulation requires patients to be positioned precisely as planned during treatment.

Immobilization Devices: Customized immobilization devices aid in maintaining consistent patient positioning.

Benefits and Considerations: Reproducibility ensures the planned dose is delivered with high precision.

b. Treatment Fields Definition: Simulation sessions define the treatment fields, including the angles and depths of radiation beams.

Technological Advances: Three-dimensional planning allows for intricate shaping of treatment fields.

Benefits and Considerations: Ensures optimal coverage of the tumor while minimizing exposure to normal tissues.

10.2.6 Quality Assurance in Treatment Planning:

a. Plan Verification: Rigorous checks ensure the accuracy of treatment plans before actual radiation delivery.

Dosimetric Analysis: Verification through dose calculations and measurements using phantoms.

Benefits and Considerations: Prevents errors and guarantees that the planned dose is delivered as intended.

b. Continuous Adaptation: Adaptive planning allows for modifications based on changes in tumor size or patient anatomy during treatment.

Imaging During Treatment: Cone-beam CT or other imaging modalities provide real-time data for adaptive planning.

Benefits and Considerations: Maximizes precision and efficacy throughout the course of treatment.

10.2.7 Technological Advances in Treatment Planning:

a. **Intensity-Modulated Radiation Therapy (IMRT)**: IMRT optimizes dose distribution through variable intensity radiation beams.

Technological Aspects: Computer-controlled adjustments during treatment ensure precise dose delivery.

Benefits and Considerations: Enhances conformality to tumor shape, minimizing radiation to healthy tissues.

b. Image-Guided Radiation Therapy (IGRT): IGRT utilizes imaging during treatment sessions to verify and adjust the patient's position.

Technological Advances: Real-time imaging enhances accuracy and allows for immediate adjustments.

Benefits and Considerations: Reduces the risk of errors and improves overall treatment precision.

c. Proton Beam Therapy Planning: Treatment planning in proton therapy involves precise calculations to exploit the Bragg peak.

Dosimetric Considerations: Planning aims to maximize proton deposition in the tumor while minimizing exit dose.

Benefits and Considerations: Utilizes proton physics for enhanced precision and reduced toxicity.

In conclusion, treatment planning and simulation are pivotal in ensuring the success of radiation therapy for prostate cancer. The integration of advanced imaging modalities, rigorous quality assurance measures, and continuous adaptation contribute to the evolving landscape of precision medicine, enhancing treatment outcomes and improving the overall quality of care for individuals undergoing radiation therapy for prostate cancer.

10.2.8 Side Effects and Management:

a. Short-Term Side Effects: Common effects include fatigue, skin irritation, and gastrointestinal discomfort.

Management: Supportive care measures, including rest and symptom-specific medications.

Impact on Quality of Life: Generally temporary, with most side effects resolving post-treatment.

b. Long-Term Side Effects:

Potential effects include urinary changes, sexual dysfunction, and the risk of secondary cancers.

Management: Ongoing monitoring and interventions, including medications or lifestyle modifications.

Impact on Quality of Life: Varied, with advancements aiming to minimize long-term effects.

c. Psychosocial Considerations:
Addressing the emotional impact of treatment, including anxiety or depression.
Support Services: Integration of counseling services and support groups.
Impact on Quality of Life: Recognizing and managing psychosocial aspects contributes to overall well-being.

Radiation Therapy for Prostate Cancer: Extensive Exploration of Side Effects and Management

Radiation therapy is a cornerstone in the treatment of prostate cancer, effectively targeting cancer cells while aiming to preserve surrounding healthy tissues. However, like any medical intervention, it can induce side effects. This comprehensive examination delves into the nuanced aspects of side effects associated with radiation therapy for prostate cancer, covering short-term and long-term effects, their impact on quality of life, and strategies for effective management.

1. Short-Term Side Effects:
a. Fatigue: Common during and after radiation treatment, impacting energy levels.

Management: Adequate rest, proper nutrition, and moderate exercise can alleviate fatigue.

Impact on Quality of Life: Temporary and often improves post-treatment.

b. Skin Irritation: Localized skin redness or irritation may occur in the treatment area.

Management: Gentle skincare, avoiding harsh products, and following medical advice.

Impact on Quality of Life: Generally temporary and resolves with time.

c. Gastrointestinal Distress: Temporary bowel changes, including diarrhea or urgency.

Management: Dietary modifications, hydration, and medications as prescribed.

Impact on Quality of Life: Often reversible, improving post-treatment.

2. Long-Term Side Effects:

a. Urinary Changes: Irritation or changes in urinary function may persist post-treatment.

Management: Medications, pelvic floor exercises, and lifestyle adjustments.

Impact on Quality of Life: Varied, with some individuals experiencing long-term effects.

b. Sexual Dysfunction: Erectile dysfunction may occur, especially in higher doses or combined therapies.

Management: Medications, counseling, and supportive interventions.

Impact on Quality of Life: Significant and may require ongoing management.

c. Rectal Issues: Long-term rectal irritation or changes in bowel habits.

Management: Dietary adjustments, medications, and ongoing monitoring.

Impact on Quality of Life: Varied, with improvements over time for some individuals.

3. Psychosocial Impact:

a. Anxiety and Depression: A cancer diagnosis and treatment can contribute to emotional distress.

Management: Counseling, support groups, and collaboration with mental health professionals.

Impact on Quality of Life: Recognizing and addressing psychosocial aspects is crucial for overall well-being.

b. Quality of Life Considerations: Cumulative impact of side effects can influence daily life and overall satisfaction.

Management: Comprehensive supportive care, including addressing physical, emotional, and social well-being.

Impact on Quality of Life: Requires a personalized approach, focusing on individual needs and priorities.

4. Late-Onset Side Effects:

a. Radiation Fibrosis: Late tissue scarring in the treated area may occur.

Management: Symptomatic relief, including medications and lifestyle adjustments.

Impact on Quality of Life: Varies, with some individuals experiencing long-term effects.

b. Secondary Cancers: The risk of developing secondary cancers due to radiation exposure.

Management: Ongoing surveillance and early detection strategies.

Impact on Quality of Life: Requires long-term monitoring but can be manageable with timely interventions.

5. Strategies for Effective Management:

a. Multidisciplinary Care: Collaboration between urologists, oncologists, and supportive care teams.

Management: Individualized treatment plans addressing specific side effects and overall well-being.

Impact on Quality of Life: Enhances overall care coordination and patient experience.

b. Supportive Therapies: Integrating complementary therapies, such as physical therapy or acupuncture.

Management: Enhances overall well-being and may alleviate specific side effects.

Impact on Quality of Life: Personalized approaches contribute to a holistic management plan.

c. Survivorship Programs: Long-term care plans addressing post-treatment needs.

Management: Regular follow-up, monitoring, and addressing emerging issues.

Impact on Quality of Life: Empowers survivors with ongoing support and resources.

In conclusion, radiation therapy for prostate cancer is a powerful intervention with potential side effects. Effective management involves a comprehensive, patient-centered approach, addressing short-term and long-term effects through collaboration among healthcare professionals, supportive therapies, and ongoing survivorship programs. Tailoring interventions to individual needs ensures a holistic strategy, promoting the best possible quality of life for individuals undergoing radiation therapy for prostate cancer.

10.2.9 Advances in Radiation Therapy:
a. Image-Guided Radiation Therapy (IGRT): Real-time imaging during treatment sessions for enhanced precision.

Technological Aspects: Integration of imaging technologies into treatment machines.

Clinical Benefits: Improved accuracy in targeting tumors, reducing margins and potential side effects.

b. Intensity-Modulated Radiation Therapy (IMRT):
Variable radiation intensity across multiple beam angles.
Precision Planning: Computer-controlled adjustment of radiation intensity during treatment.
Clinical Benefits: Minimizing radiation exposure to healthy tissues while optimizing tumor dose.

c. Stereotactic Body Radiation Therapy (SBRT):
High doses of radiation delivered in fewer sessions.
Treatment Schedule: Typically completed in 1 to 5 sessions.
Clinical Benefits: Shorter treatment duration with comparable efficacy, especially for localized tumors.

Advances in Radiation Therapy for Prostate Cancer: A Comprehensive Overview

In recent years, significant advancements have transformed the landscape of radiation therapy for prostate cancer, offering enhanced precision, reduced toxicity, and improved treatment outcomes. This extensive exploration delves into the latest innovations and techniques, covering technological advancements, treatment delivery modalities, and evolving paradigms in the management of prostate cancer.

1. Technological Innovations:

a. **Image-Guided Radiation Therapy (IGRT):** Integrates real-time imaging during treatment delivery to ensure accurate tumor targeting.

Advantages: Enhances precision by accounting for daily anatomical variations, reducing margins, and minimizing normal tissue exposure.

Technological Aspects: Cone-beam CT, MRI-guided radiation therapy, and advanced imaging algorithms improve localization and treatment accuracy.

b. Intensity-Modulated Radiation Therapy (IMRT): Delivers highly conformal radiation doses by modulating beam intensity across multiple angles.

Advantages: Allows for precise dose sculpting, sparing critical structures while delivering escalated doses to the tumor.

Technological Advances: Volumetric modulated arc therapy (VMAT) and dynamic IMRT techniques further refine dose delivery and treatment efficiency.

c. Stereotactic Body Radiation Therapy (SBRT): Utilizes high-dose radiation delivered in a few fractions to complete treatment within a shorter timeframe.

Advantages: Offers comparable oncological outcomes to conventional fractionation with fewer treatment sessions, enhancing patient convenience and resource utilization.

Technological Aspects: Advanced motion management techniques and image guidance ensure accurate delivery despite intrafractional motion.

2. Treatment Delivery Modalities:

a. Proton Beam Therapy (PBT): Utilizes protons' unique physical properties to deliver radiation with superior dose distribution and sparing of healthy tissues.

Advantages: Reduces radiation exposure to surrounding organs, minimizing toxicity and potential late effects.

Technological Advances: Pencil beam scanning and intensity-modulated proton therapy (IMPT) refine dose conformity and enable adaptive planning.

b. Brachytherapy: Involves implanting radioactive sources directly into the prostate gland, delivering high doses of radiation locally.

Advantages: Provides excellent tumor control while minimizing radiation to adjacent tissues, preserving functional outcomes.

Technological Aspects: Real-time planning and image-guided techniques optimize seed or catheter placement, enhancing treatment precision.

3. Evolving Treatment Paradigms:

a. Hypofractionation: Investigates delivering higher doses per fraction over a shorter treatment course, exploiting prostate cancer's sensitivity to fraction size.

Advantages: Reduces overall treatment time, enhancing patient convenience, and potentially improving tumor control.

Technological Considerations: Advanced planning algorithms ensure safe dose escalation while maintaining normal tissue constraints.

b. Adaptive Radiation Therapy (ART):

Incorporates real-time imaging and plan adaptation to accommodate anatomical changes during the treatment course.

Advantages: Ensures optimal dose coverage despite prostate gland motion or volume changes, reducing the risk of underdosing the tumor or overdosing healthy tissues.

Technological Advances: On-board imaging and automated planning algorithms facilitate seamless plan adaptation throughout treatment.

4. Personalized Approaches:

a. Biomarker-Guided Therapy: Utilizes molecular markers to stratify patients based on their tumor biology and predict treatment response.

Advantages: Enables tailored treatment approaches, optimizing therapy selection, and improving outcomes while minimizing toxicity.

Technological Integration: Next-generation sequencing and multiomic profiling facilitate comprehensive tumor characterization and personalized treatment algorithms.

b. Artificial Intelligence (AI) and Machine Learning: Harnesses AI algorithms to analyze complex clinical data, predict treatment outcomes, and optimize treatment planning.

Advantages: Enhances treatment planning efficiency, automates tasks, and identifies patterns that may guide personalized treatment strategies.

Technological Integration: AI-driven treatment planning systems and predictive models improve treatment decision-making and outcomes.

In conclusion, advances in radiation therapy for prostate cancer have revolutionized treatment approaches, offering unprecedented precision, reduced toxicity, and improved outcomes. The integration of cutting-edge technologies, innovative treatment modalities, and personalized approaches heralds a new era in prostate cancer management, maximizing therapeutic efficacy while enhancing patient experience and quality of life. Continued research and technological innovation will further refine and expand the therapeutic armamentarium, ultimately benefiting patients worldwide.

Radiation therapy plays a crucial role in the multidisciplinary approach to prostate cancer treatment. The diversity of its types, precision in treatment planning, management of side effects, and ongoing technological advancements collectively contribute to improving outcomes and enhancing the quality of life for individuals undergoing radiation therapy for prostate cancer

10.3 HORMONE THERAPY

Hormone Therapy in the Treatment of Prostate Cancer

Hormone therapy, also known as androgen deprivation therapy (ADT), plays a pivotal role in managing prostate cancer by targeting the male hormones, particularly testosterone, that fuel the growth of prostate cells. This extensive exploration will delve into five key subtopics, providing an in-depth analysis of the mechanisms, indications, types, side effects, and evolving trends in hormone therapy for prostate cancer.

10.3.1 Mechanisms of Hormone Therapy:

a. Androgen Deprivation: Hormone therapy aims to reduce levels of androgens, primarily testosterone, either by inhibiting production or blocking their effects on prostate cells.

Mechanisms: Orchestrated through surgical castration, medical castration using luteinizing hormone-releasing hormone (LHRH) agonists or antagonists, and anti-androgens.

b. Prostate Cancer Cell Suppression: Deprivation of androgens halts the growth and division of prostate cancer cells.

Mechanisms: Downregulation of androgen receptors, induction of apoptosis, and suppression of cell proliferation.

Clinical Impact: Temporary reduction in tumor size and control of localized disease.

Mechanisms of Hormone Therapy in the Treatment of Prostate Cancer

Hormone therapy, also known as androgen deprivation therapy (ADT), employs various mechanisms to disrupt the growth and proliferation of prostate cancer cells, primarily by targeting the actions of androgens, such as testosterone. This comprehensive examination will delve into two key subtopics, offering an in-depth analysis of both androgen deprivation and the downstream effects on prostate cancer cells.

1. Androgen Deprivation:

a. Inhibition of Testosterone Production: One fundamental approach in hormone therapy involves reducing the production of testosterone, a key androgen that fuels the growth of prostate cancer cells.

Medical Castration: Luteinizing hormone-releasing hormone (LHRH) agonists or antagonists are employed to suppress the production of luteinizing hormone, which in turn leads to decreased testosterone production by the testicles.

Surgical Castration: Orchiectomy, the surgical removal of the testicles, achieves a similar result by eliminating the primary source of testosterone production.

Clinical Impact: Lowering testosterone levels starves prostate cancer cells of the androgen they require for growth, inducing a state of androgen deprivation.

b. Blockade of Androgen Receptors:

Mechanism: Anti-androgens act by blocking the binding of androgens, including testosterone and dihydrotestosterone (DHT), to their receptors on prostate cancer cells.

Competitive Binding: Anti-androgens compete with endogenous androgens for binding to androgen receptors, preventing the activation of pathways that drive cancer cell proliferation.

Complementary to Castration: Often used in combination with medical or surgical castration to provide a dual mechanism of androgen deprivation.

Clinical Impact: By obstructing androgen receptor activation, anti-androgens further suppress the signaling cascades that promote prostate cancer growth.

2. Downstream Effects on Prostate Cancer Cells:

a. Inhibition of Androgen Receptor Signaling:

Mechanism: Androgen receptors play a pivotal role in transmitting signals that regulate the growth and survival of prostate cancer cells.

Nuclear Translocation: Upon binding to androgens, the androgen receptor translocates to the nucleus, where it regulates the transcription of genes involved in cell proliferation.

Anti-Androgen Action: By blocking androgen receptor activation, anti-androgens disrupt this signaling pathway, impeding the transcription of genes that support cancer cell survival and proliferation.

Clinical Impact: Suppression of androgen receptor signaling contributes to the inhibition of prostate cancer cell growth and induces apoptotic pathways.

b. Induction of Apoptosis and Cell Cycle Arrest:

Mechanism: Androgen deprivation therapy triggers programmed cell death (apoptosis) and halts the cell cycle, preventing further proliferation of prostate cancer cells.

Caspase Activation: Apoptotic pathways are initiated through the activation of caspases, which orchestrate the systematic dismantling of cancer cells.

Cell Cycle Arrest: Androgen deprivation induces arrest at specific points in the cell cycle, preventing cancer cells from progressing through division.

Clinical Impact: By promoting apoptosis and arresting the cell cycle, hormone therapy contributes to the reduction in tumor size and inhibits the progression of prostate cancer.

In conclusion, hormone therapy in the treatment of prostate cancer utilizes a multifaceted approach, targeting androgen production and receptor signaling to disrupt the growth and survival of cancer cells. Understanding the intricacies of these mechanisms is crucial for clinicians and patients, providing insights into the rationale behind hormone therapy and its impact on the management of prostate cancer.

10.3.2 Indications for Hormone Therapy in the Treatment of Prostate Cancer:

Hormone therapy, also known as androgen deprivation therapy (ADT), is a cornerstone in the management of prostate cancer. Understanding the specific indications for initiating hormone therapy is crucial for clinicians in tailoring treatment plans to individual patient needs. This comprehensive examination will delve into three key aspects of the indications for hormone therapy, encompassing its role in locally advanced disease, metastatic prostate cancer, and its utilization in combination with other treatment modalities.

10.3.3 Locally Advanced Prostate Cancer:

Indications: Often used as neoadjuvant or adjuvant therapy in conjunction with radiation or after prostatectomy.

Clinical Impact: Reduces the risk of recurrence and improves overall survival rates.

Hormone therapy is a cornerstone for managing cancers that have extended beyond the prostate capsule.

a. Neoadjuvant Hormone Therapy Indications: Neoadjuvant hormone therapy is often employed before definitive treatment, such as radical prostatectomy or radiation therapy, in cases where prostate cancer has extended beyond the confines of the prostate.

Goals: Reduction of tumor size and downstaging to facilitate subsequent surgical or radiation interventions.

Clinical Impact: Neoadjuvant hormone therapy aims to enhance the effectiveness of localized treatments and improve the likelihood of achieving complete cancer control.

b. **Adjuvant Hormone Therapy**:

Indications: Adjuvant hormone therapy is utilized after localized treatments like prostatectomy or radiation therapy, particularly in cases with high-risk features.

Goals: Minimization of the risk of cancer recurrence and improvement of overall survival rates.

Clinical Impact: Adjuvant hormone therapy seeks to eradicate residual cancer cells and prevent disease progression after primary interventions.

10.3.4. Metastatic Prostate Cancer:

Hormone therapy is a standard treatment for metastatic prostate cancer.

Indications: Aimed at slowing disease progression and alleviating symptoms associated with advanced stages.

Clinical Impact: Provides palliative relief, extends survival, and enhances quality of life.

a. Initial Treatment for Metastatic Disease:

Indications: Hormone therapy is the primary treatment for metastatic prostate cancer, aiming to control disease progression and alleviate symptoms associated with advanced stages.

Goals: Suppression of androgens to halt cancer cell growth, induce tumor regression, and improve overall survival.

Clinical Impact: Hormone therapy in metastatic disease provides palliative benefits, enhancing quality of life and extending survival.

b. Salvage Hormone Therapy:

Indications: Salvage hormone therapy is initiated when prostate cancer recurs or progresses despite previous local treatments.

Goals: Delaying disease progression, managing symptoms, and extending survival in the setting of recurrent or persistent metastatic disease.

Clinical Impact: Salvage hormone therapy seeks to control cancer growth and prolong disease stability after initial localized treatments.

10.3.5. Combination Therapies:
a. Hormone Therapy with Radiation:
- **Indications**: Combining hormone therapy with radiation is indicated in cases of locally advanced or high-risk prostate cancer.
- **Goals**: Enhanced local control by sensitizing cancer cells to radiation, reducing the risk of recurrence, and improving overall outcomes.
- **Clinical Impact:** The combination approach synergistically targets cancer cells locally, increasing the likelihood of eradicating residual disease.

b. Hormone Therapy in Advanced Stages:

Indications: Hormone therapy remains a crucial component in the management of advanced stages, including recurrent or metastatic disease.

Goals: Suppressing androgens to control cancer growth, alleviate symptoms, and extend overall survival.

Clinical Impact: Combining hormone therapy with other modalities, such as chemotherapy or immunotherapy, is explored to optimize treatment outcomes and address the complexities of advanced prostate cancer.

In conclusion, the indications for hormone therapy in prostate cancer are diverse, encompassing neoadjuvant and adjuvant settings for localized disease, primary treatment for metastatic disease, salvage therapy for recurrences, and combinations with other modalities to achieve comprehensive cancer management. Tailoring hormone therapy based on the specific clinical scenario is essential to optimize outcomes and improve the overall care of individuals with prostate cancer.

10.3.6 Types of Hormone Therapy in the Treatment of Prostate Cancer:

a. Luteinizing Hormone-Releasing Hormone (LHRH) Agonists:

b. LHRH Antagonists:

c) Anti-Androgens

Hormone therapy, also known as androgen deprivation therapy (ADT), encompasses various approaches aimed at suppressing the actions of androgens, primarily testosterone, which fuel the growth and proliferation of prostate cancer cells. This extensive exploration will delve into the three main types of hormone therapy used in the treatment of prostate cancer, providing an in-depth analysis of each approach, its mechanisms of action, clinical applications, and potential side efeffects

I) Luteinizing Hormone-Releasing Hormone (LHRH) Agonists:

Overview: Synthetic analogs of LHRH that suppress testosterone production by the testicles.

Administration: Typically administered through injections, either monthly or every three to six months.

Clinical Considerations: Initial testosterone surge before suppression occurs, often mitigated with anti-androgens.

a. Mechanism of Action: LHRH agonists function by initially stimulating the release of luteinizing hormone (LH) from the pituitary gland. Continuous stimulation of LH receptors leads to downregulation and desensitization of pituitary gonadotropin-releasing hormone (GnRH) receptors, resulting in decreased secretion of LH and follicle-stimulating hormone (FSH). Reduced LH levels subsequently suppress testosterone production by the testes, leading to androgen deprivation and inhibition of prostate cancer cell growth.

b. Clinical Applications: LHRH agonists are administered via subcutaneous or intramuscular injections, typically on a monthly or three to six-monthly basis. They are indicated for both locally advanced and metastatic prostate cancer, serving as the cornerstone of androgen deprivation therapy in these settings. LHRH agonists may be used as monotherapy or in combination with other modalities such as radiation therapy or chemotherapy, depending on the disease stage and patient factors.

c. Potential Side Effects: Common side effects of LHRH agonists include hot flashes, fatigue, decreased libido, erectile dysfunction, and osteoporosis. Initial testosterone surge ("flare reaction") may occur transiently upon initiation of treatment, necessitating concomitant administration of anti-androgens to mitigate symptoms. Long-term use of LHRH agonists may also increase the risk of cardiovascular events and metabolic disturbances.

II) Luteinizing Hormone-Releasing Hormone (LHRH) Antagonists:

LHRH Antagonists:

- **Overview**: Directly block LHRH receptors, rapidly suppressing testosterone without the initial surge.

- **Administration**: Administered as injections, offering a more immediate reduction in testosterone levels.

- **Clinical Considerations**: Efficacy comparable to agonists but without the initial flare.

a. Mechanism of Action: LHRH antagonists directly block the GnRH receptors on the pituitary gland, inhibiting the release of LH and FSH without the initial surge seen with agonists. This rapid suppression of gonadotropin secretion leads to immediate reduction in testosterone levels, achieving androgen deprivation more swiftly than agonists.

b. Clinical Applications: LHRH antagonists are administered via subcutaneous injection, providing a convenient and effective means of achieving rapid androgen deprivation. They are indicated for the treatment of advanced prostate cancer, both in the metastatic and non-metastatic settings. LHRH antagonists may be used as monotherapy or in combination with other treatment modalities, offering an alternative to agonists in certain clinical scenarios.

c. Potential Side Effects: Side effects of LHRH antagonists are similar to those of agonists and include hot flashes, fatigue, sexual dysfunction, and potential bone loss. Compared to agonists, LHRH antagonists may offer a lower risk of testosterone flare, making them preferable in patients with symptomatic or advanced disease.

3. Anti-Androgens:
 - **Overview**: Block the binding of androgens to their receptors on prostate cells.

- **Administration**: Administered orally, often used in combination with LHRH agonists or antagonists.

- **Clinical Considerations:** May be prescribed as monotherapy for select cases or as part of combination therapy

a. Mechanism of Action: Anti-androgens function by competitively binding to androgen receptors on prostate cancer cells, thereby blocking the actions of endogenous androgens such as testosterone and dihydrotestosterone (DHT). By inhibiting androgen receptor signaling, anti-androgens disrupt the transcriptional activation of genes involved in cancer cell proliferation and survival.

b. Clinical Applications: Anti-androgens are administered orally in the form of tablets or capsules, offering a convenient route of delivery. They are primarily used in combination with LHRH agonists or antagonists as part of combined androgen blockade (CAB) therapy. Anti-androgens may also be prescribed as monotherapy in select cases, particularly in the setting of biochemical recurrence or localized prostate cancer.

c. Potential Side Effects: Common side effects of anti-androgens include fatigue, gastrointestinal disturbances, gynecomastia, and sexual dysfunction. Unlike LHRH agonists and antagonists, anti-androgens do not cause testosterone flare, making them suitable for use without concomitant anti-androgen therapy. Long-term use of anti-androgens may be associated with adverse effects on liver function and potentially cardiovascular health.

In conclusion, hormone therapy for prostate cancer encompasses LHRH agonists, LHRH antagonists, and anti-androgens, each offering unique mechanisms of action, clinical applications, and potential side effects. Understanding the nuances of each type of hormone therapy is essential for clinicians in optimizing treatment strategies and mitigating adverse effects while maximizing therapeutic efficacy in the management of prostate cancer.

10.3.7 Side Effects of Hormone Therapy:

a. Cardiovascular Risks: Long-term hormone therapy may increase the risk of cardiovascular issues.
Side Effects: Elevated cholesterol levels, increased risk of heart disease, and potential impact on cardiovascular health.
Management: Cardiovascular monitoring, lifestyle modifications, and collaboration with cardiovascular specialists.

b. Bone Health Complications:
 Hormone therapy can lead to bone density loss and increase the risk of fractures.
Side Effects: Osteoporosis and fractures, particularly in the hip and spine.

Management: Calcium and vitamin D supplementation, weight-bearing exercises, and bone density monitoring.

5. Evolving Trends and Future Directions:

a. Combination Therapies: Investigating the efficacy of combining hormone therapy with other targeted agents.

Trends: Ongoing clinical trials explore the use of hormone therapy alongside immunotherapy, chemotherapy, or novel androgen receptor-targeted agents.

Future Directions: Personalized treatment approaches tailored to individual tumor characteristics.

b. Duration of Hormone Therapy:

Balancing the benefits of prolonged hormone therapy with potential side effects.

Trends: Emerging data guide decisions on the optimal duration, with some cases considering intermittent therapy.

Future Directions: Ongoing research aims to define the ideal duration for different clinical scenarios.

In conclusion, hormone therapy remains a cornerstone in the multifaceted approach to prostate cancer treatment. Understanding its mechanisms, indications, types, side effects, and the evolving trends in its application provides clinicians and patients with a comprehensive perspective, contributing to informed decision-making and improved outcomes in the management of prostate cancer.

10.4 IMMUNOTHERAPY

Immunotherapy in the Treatment of Prostate Cancer:

Immunotherapy has emerged as a promising frontier in the treatment of prostate cancer, leveraging the body's immune system to recognize and combat cancer cells. This extensive exploration will delve into the mechanisms, current immunotherapeutic approaches, clinical applications, challenges, and future directions in utilizing immunotherapy for prostate cancer.

10.4.1 Mechanisms of Immunotherapy:

a. Immune Checkpoint Inhibition: Immunotherapy often involves targeting immune checkpoints, such as programmed cell death protein 1 (PD-1) and cytotoxic T-lymphocyte-associated protein 4 (CTLA-4). Inhibiting these checkpoints enhances the activation of T cells, promoting an immune response against cancer cells. Checkpoint inhibitors unleash the immune system's potential to recognize and attack prostate cancer cells.

b. Therapeutic Vaccines: Therapeutic vaccines aim to stimulate the immune system to recognize specific antigens on prostate cancer cells. Antigen-presenting cells capture cancer-specific antigens and present them to T cells, triggering an immune response against the tumor. Sipuleucel-T, an FDA-approved therapeutic vaccine, exemplifies this approach in prostate cancer treatment.

10.4.2 Current Immunotherapeutic Approaches:

a. Immune Checkpoint Inhibitors: PD-1/PD-L1 inhibitors (e.g., pembrolizumab, nivolumab) and CTLA-4 inhibitors (e.g., ipilimumab) have been investigated in clinical trials. These agents aim to unleash the immune system by blocking inhibitory signals, promoting T cell activity against prostate cancer cells. Clinical trials explore their effectiveness as monotherapy or in combination with other treatments.

b. Therapeutic Vaccines: Sipuleucel-T, an autologous cellular immunotherapy, involves harvesting a patient's immune cells, exposing them to a prostate cancer antigen, and reinfusing them into the patient. Ongoing research investigates novel vaccine strategies targeting specific prostate cancer antigens to enhance immune responses.

10.4.3. Clinical Applications:

a. Metastatic Castration-Resistant Prostate Cancer (mCRPC): Immunotherapy has shown promise in mCRPC, where conventional treatments may have limited efficacy. Pembrolizumab and nivolumab, PD-1 inhibitors, have been evaluated in clinical trials for their potential in improving outcomes in advanced prostate cancer.

b. Adjuvant and Neoadjuvant Settings: Immunotherapy is explored in combination with standard treatments, such as surgery or radiation, in the adjuvant and neoadjuvant settings. Trials aim to determine the efficacy of boosting the immune response before or after primary interventions.

10.4.4 Challenges in Immunotherapy for Prostate Cancer:

a. **Tumor Microenvironment**: Prostate cancer often features an immunosuppressive tumor microenvironment, hindering the effectiveness of immunotherapy. Strategies to modify the microenvironment and enhance immune cell infiltration are under investigation.

b. **Biomarker Identification**:

- Identifying predictive biomarkers for immunotherapy response in prostate cancer remains a challenge.

- Biomarker research focuses on understanding which patients are most likely to benefit from specific immunotherapeutic agents.

10.4.5. Future Directions:

a. Combination Therapies: The future lies in exploring combination therapies, integrating immunotherapy with other modalities like targeted therapies, radiation, or chemotherapy.

Combining different immunotherapeutic approaches may enhance efficacy and broaden the spectrum of responders.

b. Personalized Medicine: Advancements in understanding the unique molecular profiles of prostate cancers may pave the way for personalized immunotherapeutic strategies.
Tailoring treatment based on individual tumor characteristics aims to optimize therapeutic outcomes.

Immunotherapy holds promise in revolutionizing the treatment landscape for prostate cancer. While challenges persist, ongoing research and clinical trials are driving innovation, offering new hope for patients with advanced or aggressive forms of prostate cancer. The dynamic evolution of immunotherapy in prostate cancer underscores the potential for transformative changes in the way we approach and treat this complex disease.

10.5 Chemotherapy in the Treatment of Prostate Cancer

Chemotherapy, a systemic approach to cancer treatment, plays a distinct role in managing advanced or metastatic prostate cancer. This comprehensive discussion explores the principles, agents, and considerations surrounding chemotherapy for prostate cancer.

10.5.1. Principles of Chemotherapy:

a. Systemic Treatment: Chemotherapy works by targeting rapidly dividing cells throughout the body, aiming to inhibit cancer cell growth.

It differs from localized treatments, such as surgery or radiation, as it addresses cancer cells that may have spread beyond the prostate.

b. Indications: Typically considered in advanced prostate cancer scenarios, especially when the disease is no longer responsive to hormone therapy (castration-resistant prostate cancer, CRPC).

Used to manage symptoms, control disease progression, and potentially extend survival.

10.5.2. Chemotherapeutic Agents:

a. Docetaxel: A taxane chemotherapy drug commonly used in advanced prostate cancer.

Acts by disrupting microtubule function, inhibiting cell division.

b. Cabazitaxel: Another taxane chemotherapy agent, often considered in cases where docetaxel is no longer effective.

*Provides an alternative mechanism of action.

10.5.3 Combination Therapies:

a. Docetaxel and Hormone Therapy: The combination of docetaxel with hormone therapy has shown improved survival outcomes in certain patient populations.

*Demonstrates the synergy between systemic chemotherapy and androgen deprivation.

b. Sequential Approaches: Some treatment plans involve the sequential use of different chemotherapeutic agents, adapting to the evolving nature of the cancer.

10.5.4. Administration and Monitoring:

a. Intravenous Infusions: Chemotherapy for prostate cancer is typically administered through intravenous infusions. Treatment schedules and dosages are determined based on individual patient factors and response to therapy.

b. Monitoring Response: Regular monitoring, including imaging studies and blood tests, helps assess the response to chemotherapy and adjust treatment plans accordingly.

10.5.5 Side Effects and Management:

a. Hematological Effects: Chemotherapy can impact blood cell production, leading to anemia, neutropenia, or thrombocytopenia.

Supportive medications or adjustments in treatment schedules may be employed to manage these effects.

b. Gastrointestinal Issues: Nausea, vomiting, and diarrhea are common side effects.

Antiemetic medications and dietary modifications can help alleviate these symptoms.

10.5.6. Advances and Ongoing Research

a. New Agents and Combinations: Ongoing research explores novel chemotherapeutic agents and combination approaches to enhance efficacy and reduce side effects.

b. Precision Medicine: Advances in understanding the molecular landscape of prostate cancer may lead to more targeted and personalized chemotherapy regimens.

10.5.7 Patient Considerations:

a. Individualized Decision-Making: The decision to undergo chemotherapy is highly individualized, taking into account factors such as overall health, treatment goals, and patient preferences.

b. Quality of Life: Balancing the potential benefits of chemotherapy with its impact on quality of life is a crucial aspect of treatment discussions.

In conclusion, chemotherapy represents a valuable tool in the multidisciplinary approach to managing advanced prostate cancer. Its role continues to evolve with ongoing research, emphasizing the importance of individualized treatment plans and a holistic approach to patient care.

CHAPTER 11

CONCLUSION

As we conclude this comprehensive exploration of prostate cancer, it's evident that understanding the intricacies of this disease is paramount for effective management and treatment. From delving into the anatomy and physiology of the prostate to unraveling the triggers of prostate cancer onset, we've embarked on a journey of discovery, shedding light on the various risk factors, molecular mechanisms, and clinical manifestations associated with this condition.

Through meticulous diagnosis methods such as digital rectal exams, PSA testing, and prostate biopsies, healthcare professionals can accurately assess the extent of prostate cancer and tailor treatment plans accordingly. We've also delved into the importance of early detection, emphasizing the critical role it plays in preserving quality of life, improving prognosis, and facilitating a wider array of treatment options.

Furthermore, advancements in diagnostic tools such as multiparametric MRI and genetic testing have revolutionized our ability to detect and classify prostate cancer, allowing for more precise risk stratification and personalized treatment approaches. We've also explored the diverse treatment modalities available, ranging from active surveillance and curative treatments to emerging therapies and clinical trials.

Importantly, this journey has underscored the significance of patient education, empowerment, and advocacy in the fight against prostate cancer. By fostering open communication, shared decision-making, and access to supportive resources, individuals can navigate their prostate cancer journey with confidence and resilience.

As we look toward the future, it's clear that ongoing research and advancements in prostate cancer care hold promise for further improving outcomes and enhancing the quality of life for affected individuals. By continuing to collaborate, innovate, and raise awareness, we can strive towards a future where prostate cancer is not just manageable but ultimately preventable.

In closing, let us remain steadfast in our commitment to combating prostate cancer, supporting those affected by the disease, and advocating for greater awareness, research, and access to care. Together, we can empower individuals, families, and communities to face prostate cancer with courage, hope, and resilience.

www.ingramcontent.com/pod-product-compliance
Lightning Source LLC
Chambersburg PA
CBHW052141220526
45471CB00004B/1466